The AOTA Practice Guidelines Series

Occupational Therapy
Practice Guidelines *for*

Adults With Alzheimer's Disease and Related Disorders

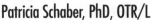

Patricia Schaber, PhD, OTR/L
Assistant Professor, Program in Occupational Therapy, Center for Allied Health Programs
University of Minnesota, Minneapolis
Member, Academy of Excellence in Scholarship of Teaching and Learning
Academic Health Center, University of Minnesota
Research Consultant, University of Minnesota Medical Center—Fairview Memory Clinic

Deborah Lieberman, MHSA, OTR/L FAOTA
Series Editor
Program Director, Evidence-Based Practice
Staff Liaison to the Commission on Practice
American Occupational Therapy Association
Bethesda, MD

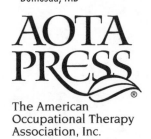

AOTA PRESS ®

The American
Occupational Therapy
Association, Inc.

Centennial Vision

We envision that occupational therapy is a powerful, widely recognized, science-driven, and evidence-based profession with a globally connected and diverse workforce meeting society's occupational needs.

Vision Statement

AOTA advances occupational therapy as the pre-eminent profession in promoting the health, productivity, and quality of life of individuals and society through the therapeutic application of occupation.

Mission Statement

The American Occupational Therapy Association advances the quality, availability, use, and support of occupational therapy through standard-setting, advocacy, education, and research on behalf of its members and the public.

AOTA Staff

Frederick P. Somers, *Executive Director*
Christopher M. Bluhm, *Chief Operating Officer*

Chris Davis, *Director, AOTA Press*
Ashley Hofmann, *Development/Production Editor*
Victoria Davis, *Editorial Assistant*

Beth Ledford, *Director, Marketing and Member Communications*
Emily Zhang, *Technology Marketing Specialist*
Jennifer Folden, *Marketing Specialist*

The American Occupational Therapy Association, Inc.
4720 Montgomery Lane
Bethesda, MD 20814
Phone: 301-652-AOTA (2682)
TDD: 800-377-8555
Fax: 301-652-7711
www.aota.org

To order: 1-877-404-AOTA (2682)

Disclaimers

This publication is designed to provide accurate and authoritative information in regard to the subject matter covered. It is sold or distributed with the understanding that the publisher is not engaged in rendering legal, accounting, or other professional service. If legal advice or other expert assistance is required, the services of a competent professional person should be sought.
—*From the Declaration of Principles jointly adopted by the American Bar Association and a Committee of Publishers and Associations*

It is the objective of the American Occupational Therapy Association to be a forum for free expression and interchange of ideas. The opinions expressed by the contributors to this work are their own and not necessarily those of the American Occupational Therapy Association.

ISBN-13: 978-1-56900-302-2
Library of Congress Control Number: 2010905196

Design by Sarah Ely
Composition by Maryland Composition, White Plains, MD
Printing by Automated Graphics Systems, White Plains, MD

Contents

Appendixes

References

Tables, Figures, and Boxes Used in this Publication

Acknowledgments

The author for this Practice Guideline is

Patricia Schaber, PhD, OTR/L

Assistant Professor, Program in Occupational Therapy, Center for Allied Health Programs, University of Minnesota, Minneapolis

Member, Academy of Excellence in the Scholarship of Teaching and Learning, Academic Health Center, University of Minnesota

Research Consultant, University of Minnesota Medical Center–Fairview Memory Clinic

The issue editor for this Practice Guideline is

Marian Arbesman, PhD, OTR/L

President, ArbesIdeas, Inc.

Consultant, AOTA Evidence-Based Practice Project

Clinical Assistant Professor, Department of Rehabilitation Science, State University of New York at Buffalo

The series editor for the Practice Guideline series is

Deborah Lieberman, MHSA, OTR/L, FAOTA

Program Director, Evidence-Based Practice

Staff Liaison to the Commission on Practice

American Occupational Therapy Association

Bethesda, MD

The author would like to acknowledge the following individuals for their contributions to the evidence-based literature review:

René Padilla, PhD, OTR/L, FAOTA

Students

Brittany Bennett, OTD, OTR/L

Kami Bogenrief, OTD, OTR/L

Kathleen Bonifer, OTD, OTR/L

Gillian Cave, OTD, OTR/L

Tessa Cooper, OTD, OTR/L

Pete Ferreri, OTD, OTR/L

Rochelle Gainer, OTD, OTR (deceased)

Erin Hiatt, OTD, OTR/L

Katie Horsager, OTD, OTR/L

Kerrie Ivey, OTD, OTR/L

Kortney Kaczmarek, OTD, OTR/L

Samuel Kim, OTD, OTR/L

Jennifer Kunsweiler, OTD, OTR/L

Miranda Materi, OTD, OTR/L

Jennifer McChesney, OTD, OTR/L

Trisha Ostrander, OTD, OTR/L

Lisa Parr, OTD, OTR/L

Ashley Sewell, OTD, OTR/L

Michelle Sierra, OTD, OTR/L

Ana Smith, OTD, OTR/L

Heather Valasek, OTD, OTR/L

Michelle Walding, OTD, OTR/L

Tracy Webb, OTD, OTR/L

Mary Worthy, OTD, OTR/L

Lori Letts, PhD, OT Reg. (Ont.)

Students

Julie Berenyi, BHSc (OT) OT Reg. (Ont.)

Mary Edwards, MHSc, OT Reg. (Ont.)

Colleen McGrath, MSc (OT), OT Reg (Ont.)

Jacqueline Minezes, MSc (RS), BSc (OT), OT Reg. (Ont.)

Kathy Moros, BHSc (OT), OT Reg. (Ont.)

Colleen O'Neill, BSc (OT), OT Reg. (Ont.)

Colleen O'Toole, MSc (OT), OT Reg. (Ont.)

The author would like to acknowledge and thank the following individuals for their participation in the content review and development of this publication:

Mary A. Corcoran, PhD, OT, FAOTA
Sharon J. Elliott, MS, OTR/L, BCG, FAOTA
Terrianne Jones, MA, OTR/L
Jana McMahon, MA, OTR/L
René Padilla, PhD, OTR/L, FAOTA
Sue M. Paul, OTR/L
Catherine Verrier Piersol, MS, OTR/L
V. Judith Thomas, MGA

The author would like to acknowledge the following institutions for their dedication to individuals and families experiencing the effects of Alzheimer's disease and support of occupational therapy in memory care:

N. Bud Grossman Center for Memory Research and Care (CMRC)
University of Minnesota Medical Center–Fairview Memory Clinic

■ ■ ■

Introduction

Purpose and Use of This Publication

Practice guidelines have been widely developed in response to the health care reform movement in the United States. Such guidelines can be a useful tool for improving the quality of health care, enhancing consumer satisfaction, promoting appropriate use of services, and reducing costs. The American Occupational Therapy Association (AOTA) represents the interests of nearly 140,000 occupational therapists, occupational therapy assistants (see Appendix A), and students of occupational therapy. AOTA is committed to providing information to support decision making that promotes a high-quality health care system that is affordable and accessible to all.

Using an evidence-based perspective and key concepts from the *Occupational Therapy Practice Framework: Domain and Process* (AOTA, 2008b), this Guideline provides an overview of the occupational therapy process for adults with Alzheimer's disease and related disorders. It defines the occupational therapy domain and process and interventions that occur within the boundaries of acceptable practice. This Guideline does not discuss all possible methods of care, and although it does recommend some specific methods of care, the occupational therapist makes the ultimate judgment regarding the appropriateness of a given intervention in light of a specific client's circumstances, needs, and available evidence to support intervention.

Through this publication, AOTA intends to help occupational therapists and occupational therapy assistants, as well as the individuals who manage, reimburse, or set policy regarding occupational therapy services, understand the contribution of occupational therapy in treating adults with Alzheimer's disease and related disorders. This Guideline also can serve as a reference for health care professionals, health care facility managers, education and health care regulators, third-party payers, and managed care organizations. Selected diagnostic and billing code information for evaluations and interventions is provided in Appendixes B and C.

This document may be used in any of the following ways:

- To assist occupational therapists and occupational therapy assistants in communicating about their services to external audiences
- To assist other health care practitioners, case managers, families and caregivers, and health care facility managers in determining whether referral for occupational therapy services would be appropriate
- To help third-party payers determine the medical necessity for occupational therapy
- To aid health and education planning teams in determining the need for occupational therapy
- To assist legislators, third-party payers, and administrators in understanding the professional education, training, and skills of occupational therapists and occupational therapy assistants
- To assist program developers, administrators, legislators, and third-party payers in understanding the scope of occupational therapy services
- To support program evaluators and policy analysts in this practice area in determining outcome measures for analyzing the effectiveness of occupational therapy intervention
- To assist policy, education, and health care benefit analysts in understanding the appropriateness of occupational therapy services for adults with Alzheimer's disease
- To help policymakers, legislators, and organizations understand the contribution occupational therapy

can make in program development and health care reform for people with Alzheimer's disease

- To support occupational therapy educators in designing appropriate curricula that incorporate the role of occupational therapy in Alzheimer's disease.

The introduction to this Guideline continues with a brief discussion of the domain and process of occupational therapy. This discussion is followed by a detailed description of the occupational therapy process for Alzheimer's disease, including a summary of evidence from the literature regarding best practices adults with Alzheimer's disease. Although this guideline was written specific to Alzheimer's disease, approaches and interventions may be applicable to other related disorders. The term *Alzheimer's disease and related disorders* is used to include those brain diseases that may be presented concurrent with Alzheimer's or undistinguishable from Alzheimer's disease (Schneider, Arvanitakis, Bang, & Bennett, 2007). In this publication, *Alzheimer's disease* will be the general term used; it may include other dementias such as Lewy bodies.

Finally, Appendix D contains a description of evidence-based practice as it relates to occupational therapy and the process used to conduct the evidence-based practice review related to Alzheimer's disease. All studies identified by the review, including those not specifically described in this section, are summarized in the evidence tables in Appendix E. Readers are encouraged to read the full articles for more details.

Domain and Process of Occupational Therapy

Occupational therapy practitioners'[1] expertise lies in their knowledge of occupation and of how engaging in occupations can be used to support health and participation in home, school, the workplace, and community life (AOTA, 2008b).

In 2008, the AOTA Representative Assembly adopted the *Occupational Therapy Practice Framework: Domain and Process, 2nd Edition* (AOTA, 2008b). Informed by the first edition of the *Occupational Therapy Practice Framework: Domain and Process* (AOTA, 2002), the previous *Uniform Terminology for Occupational Therapy* (AOTA, 1979, 1989, 1994), and the World Health Organization's *International Classification of Functioning, Disability, and Health* (*ICF*; WHO, 2001), the *Framework* outlines the profession's domain and the process of service delivery within this domain.

Domain

A profession's *domain* articulates its sphere of knowledge, societal contribution, and intellectual or scientific activity. The occupational therapy profession's domain focuses on helping others participate in daily life activities. The broad term that the profession uses to describe daily life activities is *occupation*. As outlined in the *Framework*, occupational therapists and occupational therapy assistants[2] work collaboratively with people, organizations, and populations (clients) to engage in everyday activities or occupations that they want and need to do in a manner that supports health and participation (see Figure 1). Using occupational engagement as both the desired outcome of intervention and the intervention itself, occupational therapy practitioners are skilled at viewing the subjective and objective aspects of performance and understanding occupation simultaneously from this dual, yet holistic, perspective. The overarching mission to support health and participation in life through engagement in occupations circumscribes the profession's domain and emphasizes the important ways in which environmental and life

---

[1]When the term *occupational therapy practitioner* is used in this document, it refers to both occupational therapists and occupational therapy assistants (AOTA, 2006).

[2]Occupational therapists are responsible for all aspects of occupational therapy service delivery and are accountable for the safety and effectiveness of the occupational therapy service delivery process. Occupational therapy assistants deliver occupational therapy services under the supervision of and in partnership with an occupational therapist (AOTA, 2009).

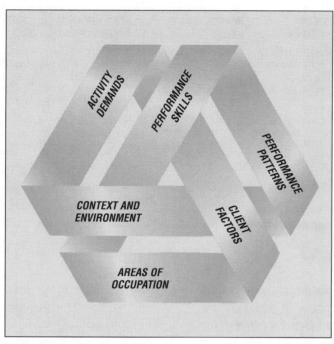

Figure 1. Domain of occupational therapy.

Note. Mobius originally designed by Mark Dow. Used with permission.

Source: American Occupational Therapy Association. (2008). Occupational therapy practice framework: Domain and process (2nd ed., p. 627). *American Journal of Occupational Therapy, 62,* 625–683. Used with permission.

circumstances influence the manner in which people carry out their occupations. Key aspects of the domain of occupational therapy are defined in Figure 2.

Process

Many professions use the process of evaluating, intervening, and targeting outcomes as outlined in the *Framework.* Occupational therapy's application of this process is made unique, however, by its focus on occupation (see Figure 3). The process of occupational therapy service delivery typically begins with the *occupational profile*—an assessment of the client's occupational needs, problems, and concerns—and the *analysis of occupational performance*—the skills, patterns, contexts and environments, activity demands, and client factors that contribute to or impede the client's satisfaction with his or her ability to engage in valued daily life activities. Therapists then plan and implement intervention using a variety of approaches and methods in which occupation is both the

means and ends (Trombly, 1995). Occupational therapists continually assess the effectiveness of the intervention and the client's progress toward targeted outcomes. The *intervention review* informs decisions to continue or discontinue intervention and to make referrals to other agencies or professionals.

Occupational therapy outcome goals may be restorative or compensatory. *Restorative intervention* seeks to change internal factors in a person that affect performance in areas of occupation. Intervention focuses on attaining restorative goals when the client shows the potential and desire for change in body functions, performance skills, or patterns of performance. Restorative intervention includes the use of selected therapeutic procedures designed to promote recovery or change in body functions, such as muscle strength or cognitive ability. Restorative intervention also includes therapeutic practice to improve performance skills and performance patterns. *Compensatory interventions* include adaptations to

AREAS OF OCCUPATION	CLIENT FACTORS	PERFORMANCE SKILLS	PERFORMANCE PATTERNS	CONTEXT AND ENVIRONMENT	ACTIVITY DEMANDS
Activities of Daily Living (ADL)*	Values, Beliefs, and Spirituality	Sensory Perceptual Skills	Habits	Cultural	Objects Used and Their Properties
Instrumental Activities of Daily Living (IADL)	Body Functions	Motor and Praxis Skills	Routines	Personal	Space Demands
Rest and Sleep	Body Structures	Emotional Regulation Skills	Roles	Physical	Social Demands
Education		Cognitive Skills	Rituals	Social	Sequencing and Timing
Work		Communication and Social Skills		Temporal	Required Actions
Play				Virtual	Required Body Functions
Leisure					Required Body Structures
Social Participation					
*Also referred to as *basic activities of daily living (BADL)* or *personal activities of daily living (PADL)*.					

Figure 2. Aspects of occupational therapy's domain.

Source: American Occupational Therapy Association. (2008). Occupational therapy practice framework: Domain and process (2nd ed., p. 628). *American Journal of Occupational Therapy, 62,* 625–683. Used with permission.

activity demands and the performance environment that enable a client to resume performance of valued occupations even when deficits in body functions, performance skills, or performance patterns are not amenable to change. Compensatory intervention approaches also involve teaching the client skills and strategies that enable him or her to use preserved abilities to work around impairments. By modifying the task demands, pattern of performance, or environment, the client may be able to continue to engage in valued occupations.

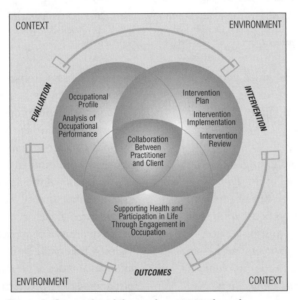

Figure 3. Occupational therapy's process of service delivery as applied within the profession's domain.

Source: American Occupational Therapy Association. (2008). Occupational therapy practice framework: Domain and process (2nd ed., p. 627). *American Journal of Occupational Therapy, 62,* 625–683. Used with permission.

Overview of Dementia— Alzheimer's Type

Dementia is an umbrella term for a constellation of symptoms that affect intellectual function. The cognitive functions are affected, causing memory impairments, along with aphasia, apraxia, agnosia, and loss of executive function (American Psychiatric Association [APA], 2000). *Aphasia* commonly manifests as word-finding difficulty; *apraxia* with motor-planning problems; *agnosia* with inability to recognize objects and their use; and *executive function loss* with planning, attention, and dexterity issues in task completion. With these symptoms, impairments in social or occupational performance characterize a decline from previous function. These impairments are beyond normal, age-related changes in cognition or functional performance and occur in the absence of a delirium, Axis I disorder (e.g., schizophrenia, depression), or other organic condition (see Table 1).

There are numerous types of dementia; some are rare but others are reaching alarming proportions. The most prevalent dementia-related diseases are Alzheimer's, which accounts for 70% of all dementias in people ages 71 or older, and vascular or multi-infarct, which accounts for 17% of dementias in people ages 71 or older (Plassman, et al., 2007).

Other diseases, including dementia with Lewy bodies, frontotemporal dementias, Huntington's, Parkinson's, amyotrophic lateral sclerosis, multiple systems atrophy, and AIDS-related dementia, account for the remaining percentages (Goetz, 2003). In addition, these related disorders have symptoms that require attention and are specific to the diagnosis (e.g., Parkinson's and motor involvement, frontotemporal dementia and self-awareness of disability, dementia with Lewy bodies and hallucinations).

Dementia is distinguished from *mild cognitive impairment,* a diagnosis that displays as minor changes in memory that interfere with managing instrumental activities of daily living (IADLs). Mild cognitive impairment is thought to be an early stage of dementia. Caselli, Beach, Yaari, and Reiman (2006) found that 10% to 15% of individuals diagnosed with mild cognitive impairment progress to dementia of the Alzheimer's type every year.

Alzheimer's Disease

Alzheimer's is an age-related, progressive, irreversible disease. The disease is named after Alois Alzheimer

Table 1. *DSM–IV* Criteria for Dementia (APA, 2000)

A. *Characteristic symptoms:* Criterion A1 must be present with one or more of Criterion A2.   – *Criterion A1:* Memory impairment   – *Criterion A2:* Aphasia, apraxia, agnosia, and loss of executive function
B. *Social/occupational dysfunction:* Criterion A1 and A2 must be severe enough to cause a significant impairment in social or occupational functioning.
C. There must be a decline from previous function.
D. The cognitive deficits are not exclusively in the course of a delirium.
E. The cognitive disturbances are not caused by another Axis I disorder (e.g., major depression, schizophrenia).

(1864–1915), a German neurologist who first identified symptoms of the disease in the last century. These symptoms were formerly classified as presenile or senile dementia or organic brain syndrome. In Alzheimer's disease, onset is insidious, and progression is gradual. The etiology is unknown, although numerous theories have been examined, including genetic mutation, neurotransmitter deficits, toxicity and environmental exposure, autoimmune processes, diet, and lifestyle (Abraham, 2005). Although the two highest risk factors are age and having a family member with the disease, more than 98% of all cases of Alzheimer's disease have no apparent genetic or familial link (Goldman, 2004). The exceptions to this statement are in Down syndrome and families of Volga-German heritage where genetic connections have been found (Goldman, 2004). The incidence of Alzheimer's disease increases exponentially over the critical age of 80 years. There is a 1.5% average risk for 80 year olds, 3.0% for 85 year olds, and 6.0% for 90 year olds (Brookmeyer, Ziegler-Graham, Johnson, & Arrighi, 2007). The prevalence is constant worldwide, with 1 in 85 people predicted to have the disease by 2050, for a total of 107 million people globally (Brookmeyer, et al., 2007). The incidence of dementia is gender influenced, with more than 30% of women and 20% of men developing it during their lifetime (Ott, Breteler, van Harskamp, Stijnen, & Hofman, 1998). The gender influence may be related to women's greater longevity.

Alzheimer's disease is progressive and ultimately fatal. The rate of progression is gradual (5 to 15 years) and consistent over time. Progression can be determined by the rate of decline from the first noticeable symptoms. The disease moves through relatively predictable stages, with characteristic symptoms present in each stage. The Alzheimer's Association has identified seven stages of the disease with descriptions of each stage (see Table 2).

The irreversible nature of the disease aligns with the other types of dementia in which reversal of symptoms is rare. Clarfield (2003) found that fewer than 0.6% of potentially reversible dementias showed any signs of improvement when the cause was treated.

Alzheimer's is a brain disease with neuropathological changes in brain tissue; a definitive diagnosis of Alzheimer's disease can be made through autopsy. Research has focused on an excessive presence of amyloid (neurotic) plaques being the hallmark pathological feature (Kelley & Minagar, 2004). However, this feature and others, such as neurofibrillary tangles, granulovacuolar degeneration, and loss of cortical neurons, are present in other neurological conditions. A relatively accurate diagnosis is made through a comprehensive

Table 2. Stages of Alzheimer's Disease (Alzheimer's Association, 2009c)

Stage 1: No impairment (normal function)
Stage 2: Very mild cognitive decline (normal age-related changes or earliest signs of Alzheimer's disease), initial lapses in memory (e.g., forgetting familiar names or location of items)
Stage 3: Mild cognitive decline (early-stage Alzheimer's); notable impairment of executive function, planning, and organizing that is apparent to family and friends
Stage 4: Moderate cognitive decline (mild or early-stage Alzheimer's disease); complex instrumental activities of daily living (IADLs) are challenging; memory lapse of recent events
Stage 5: Moderately severe cognitive decline (moderate or mid-stage Alzheimer's disease); monitoring of activities of daily living (ADLs); memory lapse of personal details, address, or phone number
Stage 6: Severe cognitive decline (moderately severe or mid-stage Alzheimer's disease); assistance needed with ADLs; tendency to wander; memory lapse of family names
Stage 7: Very severe cognitive decline (severe or late-stage Alzheimer's disease); total assistance is needed with feeding, toileting, and mobility; generally nonverbal

Note. For full descriptions of the stages of the disease, go to www.alz.org/alzheimers_disease_stages_of_alzheimers.asp

medical evaluation, which includes a history of symptoms; clinical evaluation to rule out other causes of memory impairment; radiological tests such as magnetic resonance imaging; laboratory tests to rule out metabolic disturbances, infections, or HIV; neuropsychological tests; and cognitive functional assessments. Researchers are exploring methods for earlier and more accurate diagnosis of the disease using cerebrospinal fluid biomarkers, imaging the hippocampal region (de Leon & Klunk, 2006), and magnetoencephalography imaging tracking magnetic brain wave patterns (Hua et al., 2008).

Currently, the most common screening tools used for diagnosing cognitive impairment are the Mini-Mental Status Examination (MMSE; Folstein, Folstein, & McHugh, 1975) or Cognistat (Drane et al., 2003). Neuropsychological testing can determine the nature and extent of the cognitive impairments (Lezak, Howieson, & Loring, 2004). A cognitive functional assessment is used to predict functional capacity and the need for assistance with daily activities (Baum, Morrison, Hahn, & Edwards, 2003; Burns, Mortimer, & Merchak, 1994; Rogers, Holm, Chisholm, Raina, & Toto, 2008). In the medical evaluation for Alzheimer's disease, a concerted effort should be made to distinguish the symptoms from delirium, a temporary confusional state, and depression, a mood disorder.

There is no cure for Alzheimer's, but pharmacological interventions have been reported to slow the progression of cognitive decline in 30% to 50% of patients (Moore & Jefferson, 2004).

Classification of Alzheimer's disease is based on age of onset and the presence of behavioral disturbances. *Early onset,* now termed *younger onset* by the Alzheimer's Association (2009a), is the presence of symptoms before age 65; *late onset* occurs after age 65. Although the most notable initial behaviors are short-term memory difficulties, behaviors can range from confusion, agitation, and getting lost in the early stages to delusions and confabulations, aggression, wandering, and catastrophic reactions in the later stages of the disease.

Impact of Alzheimer's Disease

Alzheimer's disease affects the person, the family, and his or her daily occupations. The effects on the person during the early stage of the disease include cognitive changes such as declines in memory, orientation, information processing, problem solving, judgment, sequencing of tasks, and object recognition (Abraham, 2005). Some people with Alzheimer's disease have relatively good motor skills, including posture, mobility, coordination, strength, and energy, well into the mid stage of the disease, whereas others show early motor involvement. Communication deficits are unique to each person with dementia. Some people experience word-finding problems as a first symptom of the disease, whereas others remain articulate into later stages of the disease. In the middle stages of the disease, the person with Alzheimer's disease may experience perceptual deficits; disorientation to person, place, and time; inability to recognize familiar faces or environments; and hallucinations or delusions. In the later stages of the disease, apraxia may cause problems with motor planning, an unsteady gait, and an increased risk for falls. By the end stages of the disease, communication is minimal, and the person with Alzheimer's disease may have difficulty eating or swallowing.

Fatigue is a problem in the middle to later stages as the person with Alzheimer's disease experiences decreased energy required to continue daily tasks. This energy lapse may be related to agitation during nighttime hours and disruption of the sleep–wake cycles characterized in approximately 25% of people with Alzheimer's disease (Bliwise, 2004). Nocturnal wandering may lead to a disruption in the sleep of the primary caregiver.

The impact on the family includes role changes. The person with Alzheimer's disease who was the primary decision maker may shift into a care receiver, necessitating a role change among family members. Family members, for the most part, take on the responsibilities of caregiving and adjust their lives to meet the supervisory challenges of care. They need to learn new skills to manage difficult behaviors, including repeated questioning, arguing or inaccurate reasoning, social withdrawal, agitation, refusals, wandering, or ultimately aggression or catastrophic reactions (Bimesser, 1997).

The impact on daily occupations entails a gradual loss of participation in work or volunteer endeavors, leisure pursuits, social interactions, and daily activities. In the early stages of the disease, minor errors in performance require monitoring, with gradually increasing supervision and assistance. As the condition progresses, daily activities become increasingly difficult to execute. Initially, in the early stage of disease, performance in the instrumental activities of daily living (IADLs) is compromised. *IADLs* are those activities "important for maintenance in a specific environment" (Gelinas, Gauthier, McIntyre, & Gauthier, 1999, p. 479). IADLs are "activities to support daily life within the home and community that often require more complex interactions than self-care used in ADLs" (AOTA, 2008b, p. 631). These include care of others, care of pets, and child care; communication management, such as telephones and emergency systems; community mobility; shopping; financial management; health management and maintenance, including scheduling appointments and administering medications; home management; meal preparation and clean up; religious observance; and safety and emergency maintenance (AOTA, 2008b).

In the middle stage of the disease, *ADLs,* or those activities important for self-care, require supervision and assistance. These include bathing or showering, bowel and bladder management, dressing, eating, feeding, functional mobility, personal device care, personal hygiene and grooming, sexual activity, and toilet hygiene (AOTA, 2008b). An aversion to bathing appears to be a common symptom and, often, the first activity with which family members need assistance. The impact of Alzheimer's disease on occupations is critical in determining supportive living situations. Two predominant reasons for ending informal caregiving and for residential transition to an institutional setting are assistance with more than three ADLs and managing challenging behaviors (Kasper, Steinbach, & Andrews, 1990).

The risk of occupational deprivation increases as the disease progresses. To promote quality of life for a person with declining cogitative abilities, work, community mobility, leisure, and recreational activities need to be altered, structured, initiated, encouraged, and supported. For example, the transition from driver to passenger imposes a change often met with resistance, despair, and altered roles for clients and their families. Social activities gradually diminish as people have increasing difficulty navigating beyond acutely familiar environments and communicating with family and friends. In the latter stages of the disease, social circles are often reduced to immediate family members.

Public health issues are related to the increase in Alzheimer's disease in the population. Elder mistreatment or abuse and neglect by the care provider increases with cognitive impairment (Dyer, Pavlick, Pace-Murphy, & Hyman, 2000). Public concerns about driving are an increasing concern, along with the appropriate timing of relinquishing this essential life skill. Studies show that drivers with early stage Alzheimer's disease had significantly more errors in driving (Uc, Rizzo, Anderson, Shi, & Dawson, 2004). Errors were related to components of cognition, including visual perception, processing, attention, verbal and visual memory, and executive functions that are affected by Alzheimer's disease (Uc, et al., 2005).

The cost of care and the emotional stress of caregiving can have a devastating impact on social programs and families (Fillit & Hill, 2005). Alzheimer's disease is the third most expensive health care condition (behind cardiovascular disease and cancer; Kirschstein, 2000), with direct and indirect costs estimated at $148 billion annually (Koppel, 2002; Lewin Group, 2004).

Prevention and Intervention

There is no definitive prevention for Alzheimer's disease, although numerous studies examine lifestyle choices that potentially delay onset or progression of the disease in early stages of the disease. Bennett and colleagues (2003) found that a person's level of education decreased the impact of Alzheimer's pathology on cognitive function. Body mass index or obesity has an effect on decline in cognition that is a contributing factor to dementia (Buchman, 2006). Metabolic disease appears to be associated with Alzheimer's in elderly patients. Researchers found that people with metabolic syndrome (high waist circumference, cholesterol, blood pressure, body mass index, and fasting glucose level) had an increased risk for Alzheimer's disease (Vanhanen, 2006). Accordingly, lifestyle behaviors that counteract metabolic disease may affect cognitive performance. Although nutritional preventative measures such as consumption of wine; Vitamins C, E, B6, B12; antioxidants; teas; and fish have been explored to reduce the risk or incidence of Alzheimer's disease, none are definitively conclusive (Luchsinger, 2004). The types of foods consumed by people with Alzheimer's disease have been found to affect disease progression. The Mediterranean diet, which includes a high intake of vegetables, legumes, fruits, cereals, olive oils, and fish, was found to reduce mortality risk affecting the course of disease (Scarmeas, Luchsinger, Mayeux, & Stern, 2007). Increased physical activity at midlife (Rovio et al., 2005) and lower cholesterol (Shobab, 2005) have been associated with lower incidence of the disease. Other lifestyle behaviors, specifically leisure activities, appear to affect the risk of dementia, with physical activity or exercise decreasing the risk of dementia (Rovio et al., 2005; Verghese et al., 2003) and boosting physical and emotional health after a diagnosis of Alzheimer's disease (Mahendra, 2004).

The goal of medical intervention for people with Alzheimer's disease is to delay the onset of symptoms, slow progression of the disease, manage challenging behaviors, and maintain quality of life. The consensus approach to treatment is interprofessional and includes pharmacologic treatment, caregiver education, behavior management, and environmental modification (Rayner, O'Brien, & Shoenbachler, 2006). Acetylcholinesterase inhibitors or donepezil (Aricept), rivastigmine (Exelon), and galantamine (Razadyne) are the drugs of choice for Alzheimer's disease (Abramowicz, 2007). Caregiver education is provided by occupational therapy practitioners, family therapists, nurses, and social workers. In the middle to later stages of the disease, behaviors may be managed using psychotropic medications and behavior

management programs. Occupational therapists design behavior management strategies that minimize disruptive behaviors to ease the burden of care for the caregiver. With the progressive nature of the disease, in the middle to later stages, a change of environment or residence may be needed to provide supports required for safety and supervision. Adult day services provide daytime respite for caregivers. Supportive living situations are available in a range of options, including group homes, assisted living facilities, memory care units, or long-term care secured units. Institutional or long-term care is the primary cost factor, consuming 92% of the total cost for care in late stages of the disease (Brookmeyer, 2006).

An occupational therapy evaluation can inform decision makers about the need and level of supportive services at each stage of the disease. Current occupational therapy practice with clients with Alzheimer's disease and their caregivers is largely based on the knowledge and clinical judgment of the treating therapist, because evidence supporting the effectiveness of any particular intervention is limited. The intervention review process, based on careful observation of client response to intervention and tracking and analysis of client progress, can contribute to the science of Alzheimer's disease intervention by providing replicable case examples. Therapists select outcome measures that are valid, reliable, and appropriately sensitive to the client's occupational performance, satisfaction, adaptation, role competence, health and wellness, prevention, self-advocacy, quality of life, and occupational justice (e.g., access to and opportunities for participation in the full range of meaningful and enriching occupations afforded to others within the community to satisfy personal, health, and societal needs [Wilcock, 2005]). Maintaining quality of life with a progressive condition includes promoting optimal participation in daily activities. Occupational therapy services are provided to maximize engagement in day-to-day leisure, social, life-skill, and self-care activities.

Family-Centered Care Models

Families are the primary caregivers for family members with Alzheimer's disease. The Alzheimer's Association (2009a) reported that in 2008, 9.9 million family members, friends, and neighbors provided informal or unpaid care. Women provide 72% of the unpaid services for caring for a spousal family member (Jecker, 2001) and 60% of unpaid services for relatives and nonrelatives (Alzheimer's Association and National Alliance for Caregiving, 2004). The amount of care increases as the disease progresses and with the impact of co-occurring diagnoses. Eventually, in the middle to later stages of the disease, 24-hour supervision is needed because of exiting or sensory-seeking behaviors. Many people with Alzheimer's live at home through the middle stage of the disease until disturbances in sleep patterns or incontinence overwhelm the primary caregiver.

With clients who are dependent on family members for care, the model for intervention is family centered (Corcoran, 1999). The *family-centered* model situates the person within the context of the family and includes family members in determining treatment approaches and outcomes (Lawler & Mattingly, 1998). Beyond consideration of the client's needs, a family-centered care model takes into account the caregiver's needs, including physical and emotional demands of providing care. With Alzheimer's disease, family members serve in various roles, acting as informant in the initial stages to provide information about the client's occupational performance and need for services. As the disease progresses, family members may act as case managers guiding treatment decisions, therapy aides modifying the environment, team collaborators in planning interventions, or co-recipients of care through family education about the disease (Brown, Humphry, & Taylor, 1996).

Family members, as primary caregivers, serve increasingly as proxies and decision makers as the person with Alzheimer's disease relinquishes decision-making roles. Family members have been referred to as the hidden client in the therapist–client dyad (Shaw, Kearney, Vause Earland, & Eckhardt, 2003). They provide information to identify the barriers and supports for occupational participation, adapt the environment, adjust the activity demands, and guide compensatory strategies. With the continual change in client abilities and related family roles, interventions in the form of caregiver education need to specifically address the challenges of family life with Alzheimer's disease (Garwick, Detzner, & Boss, 1994). In a family-centered care model, therapists need to be cognizant of the distress spousal caregivers experience and the effect on their emotional involvement with one another (Blieszner, Roberto, Wilcox, Barham, & Winston, 2007). Training families in problem-solving and trial-and-error approaches to solutions help caregivers face the uncertainty of the disease. Negotiation and conflict resolution skill development has been found to have a positive effect on family cohesion and the outcomes of intervention (Gwyther, 1995).

Occupational therapy is an integral service in the team approach to the diagnosis, management, and treatment of people with Alzheimer's disease. The goal of occupational therapy is to maximize quality of life through optimal engagement in daily activities. The burgeoning population of people with Alzheimer's disease and families facing the care of a family member with this disease generates a challenge for the health care system and an opportunity for occupational therapy professionals to meet this challenge. This guideline will examine the occupational therapy process in the treatment of people with Alzheimer's disease.

■ ■ ■

Occupational Therapy Process for Adults With Alzheimer's Disease

Setting for Service Delivery

Occupational therapy services for people with Alzheimer's disease are provided in multiple settings, depending on the service delivery model. In the early stages of the disease, the occupational therapy practitioner provides services in a hospital, transitional care unit, specialized memory clinic, outpatient clinic, community agency, adult day service program, or home care setting. Client and caregiver education is provided in all settings and continues even after the individual is transitioned to residential placement. The occupational therapy process encompasses areas of occupation, performance skills and patterns, context and environmental influences, activity demands, and client factors in a family-centered care model during the process of making recommendations for a residential change. Occupational therapy practitioners provide services in residential facilities, including assisted living, memory care, and skilled nursing facilities. Residential placement recommendations are made in conjunction with information provided by the health care team.

Occupational therapy practitioners deliver services in community settings using a direct-service or a consultative approach or through program administration. These settings may be adult day services, adult foster care, adult respite care, assisted living facilities, community centers, or programs that serve seniors with special needs. The services may be consultative for an individual or on a programmatic level. In addition, occupational therapists may be administering, directing, or coordinating programs for private or public agencies or organizations that serve people and families managing dementia care.

Many people with Alzheimer's disease can live in their home for years because of the gradual and slow progression of the disease, especially if there is a caregiver who is available most of the day (Alzheimer's Association, 2009a). Supportive services such as personal care attendants or adult day services are designed to provide supervision and adapted activities for people with cognitive deficits. These services provide caregiver respite or reprieve from the continual demands of care. If a residential change is necessary, memory care facilities, or skilled nursing facilities provide up to 24 hours of supervision per day. Often, a change in residence occurs because of unavailable family caregivers or client factors of incontinence, altered sleep–wake cycles, or behavior management problems. In the later stages of the disease, a skilled nursing facility or dementia unit is needed to ensure safety and proper medical care.

Family Collaboration

When a family member has Alzheimer's disease, it affects all family members, especially those who provide the ongoing support and care. For this reason, the term *families with Alzheimer's disease* is used in this Practice Guideline. The needs of a client as a family member include the need to belong, the need to have decisions made for him or her and reassurance about the decisions, and the need for affection (Schaber, 2002). Families, for the most part, may naturally adapt to meet these needs but may benefit from the guidance of the occupational therapy practitioner in adapting activities for enhanced participation. An occupational therapy evaluation includes an informal assessment of social support to determine the primary and secondary caregivers who may collaborate in the intervention plan.

Occupational Therapy Process

Occupational therapy has been demonstrated as effective in managing the occupational performance of people with Alzheimer's disease (Gitlin, Hauck, Dennis, & Winter, 2005; Graff et al., 2006). The occupational therapy process begins with an evaluation to determine the impact of cognition on areas of occupation (IADLs, ADLs, work or volunteer, leisure, social participation, rest and sleep), performance skills (sensory perception, motor and praxis, emotional regulation, cognitive processing, communication and social skills), performance patterns (habits, routines, roles, rituals), client factors (body functions and structures, spirituality, values, beliefs), and contexts and environments (cultural, physical, social, personal, temporal, virtual; AOTA, 2008b). Evaluation includes an analysis of activity demands (objects, space, social, sequencing and timing, requires actions, body functions and structures; AOTA, 2008b). Intervention plans are designed by considering client and caregiver factors, environmental supports, and occupational goals. To facilitate occupational performance and increase participation, intervention strategies incorporate established habits and routines within a consistent physical and social context (Gitlin et al., 2005). The key to effective intervention with a person with cognitive challenges is to equalize the activity and environmental demands to the person's capabilities (Corcoran et al., 2002; Gitlin, Corcoran, Winter, Boyce, & Hauck, 2001). Interventions are monitored, reviewed, and altered to guide the individual toward targeted outcomes. Outcomes are measured, reported, and included as part of a larger, comprehensive program evaluation. The occupational therapy process necessitates the skills of an experienced clinician trained in assessment and intervention of people with dementia.

Referral

In the early stages of Alzheimer's disease, referral to occupational therapy is appropriate when an individual exhibits a decline or impairment in performance of functional activities because of problems with thinking, memory, or executive function. The individual may report general memory or communication difficulties to a health care provider, but often a family member is the one who raises concerns about occupational performance in IADLs and hazardous activities such as cooking on a stovetop, operating machinery, or getting lost when driving. These concerns are frequently echoed by adult children, employers, friends, and community members. In the early stages of the disease, a referral is indicated if cognitive limitations are barriers to participation in daily living skills, social activities, leisure interests, or work and volunteer activities. In the middle stages of the disease, additional indications for referrals may be to determine service needs such as home health assistance, memory care or day service programs, or caregiver respite support. In later stages of the disease, occupational therapy is referred to resolve barriers to performance in self-care or to manage challenging behaviors such as agitation, aggression, disruptive vocalizations, wandering, altered sleep–wake cycles, catastrophic reactions, or frustrations related to communication problems.

Referrals may be initiated by a client or a family member or may come from a physician (geriatrician, geropsychiatrist, neurologist, family practitioner), nurse (nurse practitioner, public health nurse), neuropsychologist, or social worker. The referral may indicate a specific purpose for the occupational therapy evaluation, such as cognitive performance testing for diagnostic information (for the physician, the presence of cognitive deficits that affect functional performance may discriminate mild cognitive impairment from dementia; a physician would use this information in diagnosing) or be a general order for an evaluation and intervention. For some clients, their first encounter with occupational therapy is in rehabilitation in a transitional or subacute care unit after a precipitating event, such as a fall or illness. A cognitive functional screening as part of an occupational therapy evaluation may serve as a referral for further cognitive assessment. Some specialty memory disorder clinics that use a team approach have a standing referral for clients that includes occupational therapy evaluation as an integral part of a comprehensive assessment for dementia.

Evaluation

The occupational therapy evaluation is conducted with the client, caregiver or family member, or health care proxy to facilitate an accurate exchange of information. Questions should be directed toward the client, allowing the client to take an active and central role in the interview process. Others present should be encouraged to provide additional information, if appropriate. Information is gathered through an occupational profile (interview), analysis of occupational performance (observation), and standardized and nonstandardized assessments. This section of the Guideline outlines areas for evaluation using the *Occupational Therapy Practice Framework* (AOTA, 2008b) classification and justifies the rationale as it relates to characteristics of Alzheimer's disease.

The occupational therapist obtains client information through the occupational profile to determine barriers to occupational performance. If cognition is the primary concern limiting participation, a brief cognitive assessment using a screening tool such as the Large Allen Cognitive Lacing Screen is administered to determine whether a full cognitive functional assessment is warranted (Allen et al., 2007). Some standardized cognitive functional assessments such as the Cognitive Performance Test (CPT; Burns, 2006) or the Executive Function Test (Baum et al., 2003) may require additional training to administer and interpret, reflecting a specialized area of practice.

An individual with cognitive deficits may exhibit a decline or impairment in performance of functional activities caused by comorbidities that affect motor and praxis, sensory–perceptual, emotional regulation, cognitive, communication, and social skills. One difficulty in assessment with comorbidities is delineating the source of the performance deficit. With clinical expertise, all factors that limit occupational performance are considered, along with thinking, memory, or executive function abilities. These factors need to be considered when selecting valid assessment tools. For instance, verbally based assessments may not be valid when auditory deficits are present, and perceptual tests lose validity when visual deficits are evident. Through skilled selection and administration of the assessment and interpretation of the results, the occupational therapy evaluation contributes to an individualized intervention plan.

Occupational Profile (Family/Caregiver Profile)

The occupational profile is a nonstandardized assessment to obtain background information about the client (see Table 3). It includes demographic information about the client, family members, living situation,

Table 3. Sample Occupational Profile Information

Date:
Name:
Marital status:
Gender:
Age:
Educational level:
Employment or employment history:
Diagnoses:
Mini-Mental Status Examination (MMSE):
Large Allen Cognitive Level Screening Tool–5 (lacing score):
Primary caregiver:
Offspring:
Living situation (alone, with family, house, apartment, assisted living):
Predominant concerns/family concerns:
Mobility/upper-extremity function:
Leisure and routine activities:
Family impression of cognitive involvement:
"Describe a typical day":
Safety procedures/precautions: ❑ Carries personal identification ❑ Has Life Alert system or similar alarm system ❑ Wears Life Alert system and uses appropriately ❑ Has gotten lost in familiar locations ❑ Has gotten lost in unfamiliar locations ❑ Registered with Safe Return program ❑ Uses phone for emergencies ❑ Uses appliances (e.g., stove, iron, microwave) ❑ Uses machinery (e.g., lawn mowers, snow blowers) ❑ Hunts or handles firearms ❑ Provides child care ❑ At high risk for falls (reports a previous fall)

employment or employment history, education, caregivers or people responsible for care, diagnoses including mental health diagnoses, resources, and reasons for the referral. Questions about leisure interests, strengths and limitations to participation in daily activities, and goals of intervention can be included (see Table 4). The Canadian Occupational Performance Measure is an evidence-based, standardized tool used to identify occupational performance issues and to prioritize the selection of intervention goals with client and family input (Law et al., 2005). Client and family goals are obtained to guide the family-centered intervention process.

The occupational profile includes the client and family member's description of the cognitive or memory impairments that may affect safety. Through the interview, the occupational therapist gains a sense of the client's self-awareness of disability. Self-awareness is important in making recommendations about supportive living situations and levels of assistance needed to remain safe in the home environment. Family members should be asked to describe their observation of the client's memory or thinking problems. The client's perception may differ from the family member's perception, especially in the middle to later stages of the disease, which will influence the strategies

for intervention. Observation of the client provides an opportunity to screen for client factors that may guide the appropriate selection of assessments.

An occupational history provides information regarding participation in daily activities. "Describe a typical day" is a standard question. The client will identify activities he or she is able to perform or enjoys doing and may be considered the client strengths. Often these activities are habits or routines that are well rehearsed or rote, drawn from long-term or procedural memory. An occupational history includes information about those activities the client used to do but now finds challenging. An "interest checklist" can stimulate discussion about activities the client desires to continue and barriers to participation (Kielhofner, 2008, p. 383). Attention to the amount of time the person is engaged in activities is important because of the tendency to socially isolate or sleep for lengthy periods during the day or the propensity for occupational deprivation (obstructing occupational enjoyment because of disease; Bass-Haugen, Henderson, Larson, & Matuska, 2005) in the middle to later stages of the disease.

An important part of the occupational profile is to gain information about the physical environment, or living situation, and social environment, or available caregiver support. Key to effective management of the disease is providing environmental supports for safety and optimal functioning. Clients with dementia symptoms come to an evaluation from a variety of living situations with different levels of support—from living independently in a single family home to residing in a memory care facility with 24-hour supports in place. Promotion of security is targeted to prevent the six most common household injuries: falls and slips, burns, poisoning, cuts, electrocution, and drowning (Warner, 2000). A home safety assessment such as the Home Environmental Assessment Protocol (Gitlin et al., 2002) or Safety Assessment of Function and the Environment for Rehabilitation (Letts, Scott, Burtney, Marshall, & McKean, 1998) can highlight necessary adaptations to the home to promote a safe environment and support caregiver supervisory responsibilities.

Table 4. Sample Occupational Profile Questions

1. What is your name?
2. Who did you bring with you today? (Introduce family members)
3. Where do you live?
4. Describe your living situation.
5. Are there other family members? Where do they live? How often do they visit you?
6. Are you employed? What was your primary employment?
7. Describe your memory and thinking abilities in your own words.
8. Can I ask your family members to describe what they observe to be your memory or thinking abilities?
9. Describe what you do in a typical day (the activity demands).
10. To the family member: Can you add anything to his or her typical day?
11. What do you hope to gain through this evaluation?
12. To the family member: What are your desired outcomes of this evaluation?

A significant factor in managing care throughout the course of the disease is the presence of a caregiver. A study on residential transition found the presence of potential caregivers had a statistically significant effect on the risk of transition from home to institutional placement (Waidmann, 2003). Aging in place, in which services and resources are added as needed to a person in his or her natural environment, requires the availability of adequate supports. Families with increased contact through geographic proximity, phone, mail, and e-mail have a greater propensity to provide informal family care (Tomaszewski, 2002) and promote aging in place. Family members may live geographically close but be unable to provide the supervision or assistance needed for safety and proper care. With a spousal caregiver, some clients are able to live in the community into the middle and even later stages of the disease.

Analysis of Occupational Performance

In conjunction with the occupational profile, the occupational analysis includes observations or interviews to obtain information about areas of occupation, performance skills and patterns, contexts, activity demands, and client factors. Analysis includes administration and interpretation of select standardized and nonstandardized assessments in specific performance areas where more information is needed (see Table 5 for assessments). With

Table 5. Selected Assessments of Occupational Performance for Adults With Alzheimer's Disease

Domain	Assessment
Areas of Occupation	Occupational profile
	Canadian Occupational Performance Measure (Law et al., 2005)
	Occupational Self-Assessment (Baron, Kielhofner, Iyenger, Goldhammer, & Wokenski, 2006)
Activities of daily living	Performance Assessment of Self-Care Skills (Holm & Rogers, 1999)
	Kohlman Evaluation of Living Skills (Kohlman Thompson, 1992)
	Direct Assessment of Functional Abilities (Karagiozis, Gray, Sacco, Shapiro, & Kawas, 1998)
	Functional Independence Measure (Keith, Granger, Hamilton, & Sherwin, 1987)
Instrumental activities of daily living	Routine Task Inventory (Heimann, Allen, & Yerxa, 1989)
	Lawton Scale for Instrumental Activities of Daily Living (Lawton, 1969)
	Disability Assessment for Dementia (Gélinas et al., 1999)
	Functional Activities Questionnaire (Pfeffer, Kurosaki, Harrah, Chance, & Filos, 1982)
	Scorable Self Care Evaluation (Tarbell, Henry, & Coster, 2004)
Work	Structured observation of performance of work activities
Leisure	Activity Interest Checklist (Kielhofner, 2008)
Social participation	Client/family interview
Sleep	Client/caregiver report of sleep habits
Performance Skills	
Sensory perceptual	Assessment of Motor and Process Skills (Fischer, 1997)
Motor and praxis	Assessment of Motor and Process Skills (Fischer, 1997)
	Tinetti Assessment Tool (Tinetti, 1991)
	Berg Balance Scale (Berg, Wood-Dauphinee, & Williams, 1992)
	Timed Get-Up-and-Go Test (Shumway-Cook, Brauer, & Woollacott, 2000)
	Functional Reach Test (Weiner, Cuncan, Chandler, & Studenski, 1992)
	6-Minute Walk Test (Bendall, Bassey, & Pearson, 1989)

(continued)

Table 5. Assessments of Occupational Performance for Adults With Alzheimer's Disease *(cont.)*

Domain	Assessment
Performance Skills (cont.)	
Emotional regulation	Geriatric Depression Scale (Yesavage et al., 1983)
Cognitive screening tests	Behavioral observation
Cognitive functional assessments	Large Allen Cognitive Level Screening Tool–5 (Allen et al., 2007)
	Allen Diagnostic Module (Allen & Reyner, 2008)
	Cognistat; Mini-COG (Engelhart et al., 1999)
	Mini-Mental Status Exam (Folstein et al., 1975)
	Cognitive Performance Test (Burns 2006; Burns et al., 1994)
	Kitchen Task Assessment (Baum & Edwards, 1993)
	Executive Function Performance Test (Baum et al., 2003).
	Loewenstein Occupational Therapy Cognitive Assessment (Katz, Itzkovich, Averbuch, & Elazar, 1989)
	Ross Information Processing Assessment (Ross, 1986)
	Baylor Profound Mental Status Examination (Doody et al., 1999)
	Self-Care Performance Tool (Thralow & Schauback Reuter, 1993)
Communication and social	Informal observation of interaction skills
Performance Patterns	
Habits	Occupational profile
Routines	Role Checklist (Oakley, Kielhofner, Barris, & Reichler, 1986)
Roles	Family/caregiver interview
Rituals	Family/caregiver interview
Context and Environments	
Cultural	Kawa model (Iwama, 2006)
	Occupational profile
Physical	Home Environment Assessment Protocol (Gitlin et al., 2002)
	Home Safety Evaluation (Letts et al., 1998)
Social	Family assessment—caregiver availability
Personal	Nutritional assessment
	Michigan Alcohol Screening Test (Selzer, Vinokur, & van Rooijen, 1975)
Temporal	Time configuration assessment
Virtual	Assistive technology assessment
Activity Demands	
Objects used and their properties	Observation during task performance
Space demands	Perimeters (Warner, 2000)
Social demands	Client/family interview
Sequencing and timing	Activities of daily living evaluation
Required actions	Positioning evaluation
Required body functions and structures	Falls risk evaluations
Client Factors	
Body functions	Proprioceptive and kinesthetic assessment
	Adult Sensory Profile (Brown & Dunn, 2002)
Body structures	Vision and hearing
	Strength and range-of-motion tests
Spirituality	Family/client interview

Alzheimer's disease, a key piece of the assessment process is a measure of cognitive functional abilities, or how the person draws from thinking and memory to organize and execute daily tasks.

The impact of cognition on performance skills and performance patterns must be considered in the selection and administration of standardized and nonstandardized assessments. Other client factors such as hearing acuity, visual perception, sensory processing, motor and praxis skills, or comorbidities such as chemical dependence, anxiety disorder, and depression need to be factored into the clinical reasoning process. The occupational therapist has the expertise to synthesize all evaluation results, including activity demands specific to the client, and to determine targeted outcomes of intervention (AOTA, 2008b). Because of the progressive nature of Alzheimer's disease, new learning is not the focus of the intervention; rather, caregiver education, environmental adaptations, and compensatory strategies in a family-centered care approach are recommended.

Cognitive functional assessments provide information about current capabilities and predictions about future performance in areas of occupation and needs for environmental supports. Although some cognitive assessments are verbally based or administered through client and family report, the most accurate are through direct observation of performance. The Kitchen Task Assessment is a standardized, observation-based assessment tool to measure six performance areas on a 3-point scale (0 = *independent*, 3 = *totally incapable*): initiation of task, organization, performance of steps, sequencing, judgment and safety, and completion of the task (Baum & Edwards, 1993). The assessment is portable and easily administered in a home-based evaluation.

The Cognitive Performance Test (CPT) is a standardized, performance-based, seven-task assessment that measures global cognition. The score, an average of the seven subtests, has been used to predict performance of IADLs and ADLs (Burns & Levy, 2006; Burns et al., 1994). The CPT was investigated for correlation on two measures of the Lawton, IADL

($r = .64$) and physical self-maintenance ($r = .49$; Burns, 1991, 1996). The score follows the Allen Cognitive Levels, which range from 6 = *normal* to 1 = *severely impaired*, reinterpreted for the Alzheimer's population (see Table 6). The CPT assessment also can be administered as a five-task assessment for home care evaluation (Burns, 2006).

The Executive Function Performance Test (Baum et al., 2008) is an executive function test. It was developed for people with stroke and corresponding cognitive deficits to determine their capacity to live safely and independently and the level of support they needed. It uses daily living tasks (cooking, managing medications, using the phone, paying bills) to rate a person's executive function components: initiation, organization, sequencing, safety and judgment, and completion. It rates the level of cueing required to perform the task from minimum cueing (verbal guidance) to maximum cueing (doing for the person).

Other assessments of cognition are administered by many disciplines and are verbally based. The Mini-Mental Status Exam (MMSE) can be administered by occupational therapy practitioners and is the only short cognitive screening tool recommended by the American Academy of Neurology (2008). For people presenting with relatively strong functional skills and mild cognitive impairment, a referral for neuropsychological testing is recommended. Neuropsychological testing, which measures dimensions of memory, attention, executive function, processing speed, recall, and learning, can distinguish normal aging from mild cognitive impairment or Alzheimer's disease (Kelley & Petersen, 2007).

Although cognition is the key area of assessment, other performance tasks can be assessed as part of a comprehensive evaluation with clients with Alzheimer's disease. The process scale of the Assessment of Motor and Process Skills (AMPS; Fischer, 1997) has been used to determine people's potential to live independently in the community (Kizony & Katz, 2002). The Performance Assessment of Self-Care Skills rates ADL and IADL performance in three areas: independence (amount of assist needed), safety, and adequacy (Rogers et al., 2008). The scores can guide the occupational therapist in the selection of activities for intervention

Table 6. Cognitive Performance Test (CPT) Scale of Functional Changes in Dementia

	Developed by Theressa Burns, OTR, GRECC, VA Medical Center, Minneapolis
CPT	**Characteristics of Functioning**
5.6	Normal functioning. (Absence of cognitive–functional disability.) Relevant information from all memory stores can be activated and used purposefully (executive control) to carry out complex activity with accuracy and safety.
5.0	Mild functional decline due to deficits in executive control functions (task planning, problem solving, divided attention, new learning). Difficulties may manifest in the performance of IADLs, including managing finances, job performance, driving, or following a complex medication/co-morbidity regime. Check-in support and assistance with IADLs may be needed. ADLs typically show no change.
4.5	Mild to moderate functional decline due to significant deficit in executive control functions; difficulty with divided attention and solving problems. Complex tasks are performed with inconsistency or error. With IADL, the person struggles to manage the details. ADLs may show decline in ability to self-initiate. Independent living poses significant risk for mismanagement of meals, finances, medications, and co-morbidities. Driving poses significant safety risks, with inability to divide attention to environmental cues. The family often experiences crisis point. IADL assistance and/or in-home assistance is needed. Assisted living environments may provide a good fit.
4.0	Moderate functional decline, from abstract to concrete thought processes. The person relies on familiar activities and environments and uses what they see for cues as to what to do. IADLs need to be done by or with others. ADLs are remembered, but the quality typically shows decline. The person benefits with structure and simple routines and may benefit from day services. Hazardous activities require supervision or restriction. The person is not safe to live alone.
3.5	Moderate functional decline; concrete thought processes. ADLs require set up and often direction during performance. Needs 24-hour care at this stage; may benefit from supportive residential placement.
3.0	Moderate to severe functional decline; from concrete to object-centered thought processes. Increased cues needed during tasks. One-to-one assistance for all ADLs.
2.5	Severe functional decline, from object-centered to movement-centered. Poor use of familiar objects. Total assist with ADLs. Resistant with cares. Little speech.
2.0	Severe functional decline, poor recognition of people. Intermittently responsive.
1.0	Late-stage dementia. Unresponsive to surroundings; minimal purposeful action. Comfort and hospice approach to care.

Source. Adapted from Burns, T. (2006). *Cognitive Performance Test Manual.* Pequannock, NJ: Maddak. T. Burns, GRECC VA Medical Center, Minneapolis. Reprinted with permission.

planning. The Routine Task Inventory is a rating of four areas: physical scale—ADLs, community scale—IADLs, communication scale, and work readiness scale (Katz, 2006). The score, obtained on the basis of observation or self- or caregiver report of assistance required, uses the Allen 6-point scale (6 = *independent*, 1 = *total assistance*).

Additional occupational therapy assessments may be included on the basis of client co-morbidities or reported problems in target areas. With low endurance, a brief screening assessment, the 6-minute walk test, can be used to determine community mobility skills (Bendall et al., 1989). People with dementia have a higher risk of falls; a history of falls within the past year is a strong predictor of future falls (Thurman, Stevens, & Rao, 2008). A brief balance

screen, the Functional Reach Test (Weiner et al., 1992), can be used to determine risk for falls. Appropriate falls assessments like the AMPS (Fischer, 1997) or the Tinetti Assessment Tool (Tinetti, 1991) can be administered, and prevention programs can be activated. For reported driving concerns, a formal driving evaluation by trained professionals that includes an on-road driving component can determine fitness to drive for people with mild Alzheimer's disease (Man-Son-Hing, Marshall, Molnar, & Wilson, 2007).

Areas of Occupation

The purpose of an occupational therapy evaluation is to design an intervention plan to create opportunities for participation, maintain occupational performance or modify activity demands, or prevent deterioration in performance capability. The area of occupation targeted depends on the cognitive ability of the client and stage of the disease. For instance, the focus of intervention in the early stage is work or employment, if applicable, and IADL participation, whereas the focus in the middle and later stages of the disease is ADL performance. Leisure, social participation, and rest/sleep are considered through the early to the later stages of the disease.

IADLs

Early signs of Alzheimer's disease include family concerns about the client's ability to drive, manage finances, self-administer medications, or make a meal. The concerns usually stem from an incident in which the client got lost while driving to a familiar location, left a stove on, had a rapid weight loss, experienced a medical crisis because of poor medication management, or had unpaid bills because of financial mismanagement. A cognitive assessment along with client and family report on IADL performance can indicate the area of occupation for skilled intervention. For each IADL, the therapist obtains information to determine the amount of monitoring, supervision, or assistance needed to ensure safe and optimal task completion. Table 7 is a sample of the kind of information needed to make an informed recommendation and educational plan.

Driving is a complex IADL and poses ethical problems for people with Alzheimer's disease. The primary question is when to discontinue driving. Studies have found that drivers with even mild dementia are an increased safety risk (Dubinsky, Stein, & Lyons, 2000). For some clients, an increasing tendency to get lost, more than technical driving skills, needs to be considered. For person with declining abilities, the challenge will be factoring in reports of getting lost, family reports of episodic confusion, and passenger apprehension about riding with the person or transporting their children. The comprehensive driving evaluation is one tool for understanding the interplay between cognitive challenges and onroad performance. However, experts in the field grapple with making this decision based on functional performance (onroad as the gold standard) or cognitive decline reported by families and measured

by clinical tests (Hunt, Brown, & Gilman, 2010). Additional information on driving and community mobility for people with Alzheimer's can be found in Appendix F.

ADLs

An occupational therapy evaluation for the middle to later stages of the disease includes a cognitive assessment and ADL assessment. The focus of ADL assessment is on the cognitive capacity to plan, initiate, and complete the task in a safe, consistent (predictable), and efficient manner. The primary caregiver provides information about performance ability in dressing, bathing, grooming, and bowel/bladder control. In the middle stage, ability to complete the task may be present, but performance is inconsistent or inadequate. For example, a client may be able to don a sweater but may wear multilayer clothing inappropriately. In the later stages of the disease, ability to perform may be present, but behavioral concerns such as resistance or combativeness may impede task completion. This situation is especially true with bathing or showering activities. Information about sleep–rest cycles and bowel/bladder control is paramount in making informed decisions about residential settings. These two ADLs have the greatest effect on family decisions regarding home versus residential placement.

Leisure and Social Participation

A history of active engagement in physical leisure activities improves the physical and emotional health of people with Alzheimer's disease (Mahendra, 2004). With the disease, there is a gradual withdrawal from leisure activities because of an inability to perform or frustration caused by increased cognitive challenges. Activities that were formerly easy to do may now seem very difficult, which causes anxiety. The propensity for occupational deprivation exists when the activity demands are not altered to meet the changing abilities. There is a tendency to socially isolate, either because of language problems such as expressive or receptive aphasia or word-finding problems, or to hide the disease from former acquaintances. In the early stages of the disease, family members or friends need to encourage

Table 7. Client and Family/Caregiver Report: Guideline to IADL Performance

Name _____ Date of evaluation _____

Check all that apply.

Driving/community mobility:

❑ Has no physical impairments/comorbidities that would impede driving or community mobility.

❑ Drives independently in local/familiar and distant/unfamiliar areas alone.

❑ Drives independently in local/familiar areas alone.

❑ Drives with a navigator safely and competently.

❑ Drives with an apprehensive navigator.

❑ Drives, but family expresses a desire to end driving.

❑ Relinquished driving _____ years/months ago.

❑ Has gotten lost while driving.

❑ Has had an accident while driving.

❑ Safely navigates in the community independently.

❑ Uses public/other transportation (identify _____).

❑ Has gotten lost in the community.

❑ Comments: _____
_____
_____

Home management/maintenance:

❑ Has no physical impairments/comorbidities that would impede home management.

❑ Shops independently.

❑ Uses memory aids for shopping (identify _____ [lists, pick up orders, schedules]).

❑ Shops with a family member.

❑ Does laundry independently.

❑ Completes portions of laundry task.

❑ Cleans house independently: bathroom, kitchen, living room, makes bed.

❑ Completes portions of house cleaning tasks (identify_____).

❑ Vacuums independently.

❑ Has hired home cleaning aide.

❑ Has never been involved with home management.

❑ Does home maintenance tasks independently with machines (e.g., mows lawn, shovels/blows snow, blows leaves).

❑ Caregiver is apprehensive about client use of machinery (e.g., lawn mowers, snow blowers).

❑ Hires home maintenance helper.

❑ Has never been involved with home maintenance or not applicable because of living setting.

❑ Has minor errors in home management (e.g., forgetting shopping lists, laundry mishaps, inadequate cleaning, losing keys).

❑ Has significant errors in home management (e.g., hoarding food, unsafe use of appliances, leaving faucets on).

❑ Comments: _____
_____
_____

Table 7. Client and Family/Caregiver Report: Guideline to IADL Performance *(cont.)*

Health and medication management:

❑ Has no physical impairments or comorbidities that would impede medication administration.

❑ Monitors health independently.

❑ Needs assistance with medical appointments, scheduling, monitoring health.

❑ Has a complex medication regime (e.g., > 4 pills daily, diabetes).

❑ Sets up and self-administers medications independently with no reminders.

❑ Sets up and administers medications with occasional reminders.

❑ Has medications set up and administers with no reminders.

❑ Has medications set up and administers with reminders.

❑ Has medications set up and administered by another.

❑ Does not take medications.

❑ Has had errors in medication administration.

❑ Has missed appointments or untreated medical issues.

❑ Comments: _____

_____

_____

Personal finances:

❑ Has no physical impairments or comorbidities that would impede conducting personal finance management.

❑ Handles personal finances independently.

❑ Handles personal finances, but another person monitors periodically.

❑ Handles personal finances, but another person checks all transactions.

❑ Handles portions of personal finances (e.g., paying bills, debit and credit cards), but another person completes selected portions of the task.

❑ Another person handles all personal finances.

❑ Has never had the responsibility for handling personal finances.

❑ Has signed over power of attorney for finances.

❑ Has had errors in personal finance transactions (e.g., late payments, overdrafts, losing credit cards or checkbook).

❑ Has had major errors in personal finance transactions (e.g., overspending or irrational spending, multiple charities, identity theft, bill collectors).

❑ Comments: _____

_____

_____

Meal preparation:

❑ Has no physical impairments or comorbidities that would impede meal preparation.

❑ Able to prepare a complex meal independently.

❑ Able to prepare a full meal with some cues, assistance from another person.

❑ Able to prepare a light meal and portions of a complex meal.

❑ Able to make light snack.

❑ Able to assist with preparation of a meal with continual supervision.

❑ Able to serve self a snack or meal prepared by another.

❑ Has never had the responsibility of preparing food for self.

❑ Has had errors in meal prep or unsafe meal prep incidents (e.g., leaving stove on, burns, unsafe preparation).

❑ Eats out frequently (> 5 times/week).

❑ Comments: _____

_____

_____

the person with Alzheimer's disease to keep him or her engaged and to creatively adapt leisure activities successfully (Gitlin et al., 2008). In the middle to later stages of the disease, specialized programs with adapted activities, such as adult day services, provide an outlet for appropriate activity stimulation. Gathering information about former leisure interests and social groups may lead to more effective intervention planning individually tailored to the client.

Performance Skills

Sensory and perceptual skills are progressively affected throughout the course of Alzheimer's disease. Although all sensory areas may be affected (visual, auditory, tactile, proprioceptive, vestibular, olfactory, and gustatory), the deficits are particular to the individual. One client may report visual perceptual disturbances, whereas another may report an aversion to certain foods or food textures. *Astereognosis,* in which a person is unable to identify an object by touch, is not uncommon. The degree and type of sensory impairment may be related to the area of the brain most involved. For this reason, the occupational therapy practitioner needs to be aware of individual skills on a case-by-case basis. Standardized visual–perceptual assessments may lack accuracy because of confounding factors such as verbal limitations and cognitive impairments.

Some clients with Alzheimer's disease have good motor skills in the early stages of the disease unless there are comorbidities that affect motor function. They are able to handle objects and complete tasks, especially those tasks that are overlearned and performed in a familiar environment. Motor skills begin to decline in the middle stages of the disease, specifically in the areas of motor planning, sequencing, and executing new movements. For example, a person may be able to insert a key into a lock but may not know the sequence of turn key, turn knob, push door to open. Cognitive deficits impede motor function. For instance, the person may not be able to problem solve the use of different knobs to open the door. In the middle to later stages of the disease, the risk of falls increases as apraxia, or the ability to motor plan, is affected. Falls may be caused by lack of judgment

in the ability to descend a staircase, perceptual dysfunction, or failure to set the brakes on a wheelchair when transferring. Motor skills in the later stages of the disease are severely impaired, and the client may require a positioning evaluation for bed, wheelchair, or Geri-Chair.

Emotional regulation is defined as the "actions or behaviors a client uses to identify, manage, and express feelings while engaging in activities or interacting with others" (AOTA, 2008b, p. 640). Early diagnosis of Alzheimer's disease is generally accompanied with a sense of loss and grieving if the person has a self-awareness of memory loss. These emotional reactions range from mild depression to overt anger and aggression. Families may encounter increasing frustration as the person has difficulty verbalizing the experience of memory loss or expressing fears about the future. Emotional regulation is evaluated through direct observation or family/caregiver report of behaviors that may be manifesting underlying feelings of confusion. In the later stages of the disease, these behaviors may escalate to aggression or catastrophic reactions and may precipitate a residential change to a facility that is designed to manage challenging behaviors. After assessing emotional regulation, the practitioner can model or educate the caregiver in providing emotional support to the person as the disease progresses.

The primary impact in performance skills is with cognitive deficits. The evaluation includes the rate of progressive cognitive deficits based on client and caregiver report and specific components of cognition. Although the primary cognitive challenge is memory, clients lose executive function, including judgment, problem-solving ability, sequencing, organizing, prioritizing, planning, and initiating. For instance, in the middle stages of the disease, the client may be immobilized by the command "get ready for your appointment." By contrast, the caregiver may offer a coat, initiate donning, and the client will continue through completion. At each stage, cognitive deficits need to be reevaluated to determine the degree of adaptations or supports needed.

Communication and interaction skill deficits range widely among people with Alzheimer's disease. Although some people can hold a cohesive conversation into the middle stages of the disease, others lose the ability to interact early in the disease. This symptom may be manifested as receptive or expressive aphasia. Problems with word finding or recalling recent events impair the flow of conversation, and the individual may retreat from group discussions. The person may be embarrassed by the challenges and may attempt to hide the problem by withdrawing from social situations. Repeating questions or perseverating on a recent event or health problem can lead to annoyances for the primary caregiver. Evaluating communication and social interactions relies on client and caregiver report. The practitioner can gauge the client/caregiver interaction and counsel or model strategies. Effective communication requires patience on the part of the caregiver to reassure and respond multiple times with the same information.

Performance Patterns

Performance patterns are the habits, routines, rituals, and roles in daily activity. Habits become strengths that the person can draw from when he or she is no longer able to remember how to perform. Because habits are automatic, people may engage in an occupation beyond their cognitive ability to do so. A person into the middle and later stages of dementia can function optimally when he or she is able to draw from early learning in long-term memory and replicate skills that are well rehearsed. New learning is challenging with dementia. The person who is unable to learn a new routine may be able to carry out former routines successfully. People with cognitive impairment report that consistency in task demands and stability in their daily environment contributes to decreased stress and anxiety. Part of the evaluation process is to consider the person's former habits, routines, and rituals that were familiar and support occupational performance. The goal for family caregivers is to support habitual behavior and adapt routines for optimal functional performance.

Contexts and Environments

A primary focus of evaluation and intervention with a progressive, cognitive disorder is on the physical and social environment or the cultural, personal, temporal, and virtual contexts that affect occupational performance. These factors can be supports or barriers to engagement in occupation.

Physical Environment

Natural and built nonhuman environment is a key area of evaluation for occupational therapy that has the potential to affect interventions and management of the care of a person with Alzheimer's disease. Environments include the primary living space and places that the person frequents in day-to-day activities. Aging in place means that the environment can be adapted to provide the precautionary supports for safety and independence. Physical environments also include the transportation systems accessible for people with cognitive decline. A home safety or fall prevention assessment can guide recommendations for environmental changes, such as increased lighting, reflective tape on stairways, or noise reduction; a community assessment can influence strategies for alternative modes of transportation to lessen the impact of driving restrictions. Many resources are available through state and county public health agencies and the Administration on Aging (2009) to facilitate environmental adaptations.

Social Environment

The *social environment* includes people in the client's life who are able to provide supports in daily living activities. Evaluating the social supports is accomplished through interview of the client and family members. It is important to know who is the primary caregiver and decision maker and the responsibilities that person is willing to accept. The social environment includes both paid (formal) and unpaid (informal) supports. Beyond family members, friends or neighbors also may be willing to provide assistance with weekly or daily tasks. This assistance may entail a simple task like driving to a weekly card club or daily fitness center. Paid supports may range from checking on the person daily (15 min) to a live-in home health aide (24 hr). Community agencies provide an array of social services, including Meals on Wheels, grocery delivery, transportation services, county public health nursing, or church-based support. Even with strong family support, there is a basic need for belonging and human contact throughout the course of the disease (Schaber, 2002). Human contact can be provided by people trained to interact with individuals with limited verbal skills or moderate-to-severe cognitive decline. Programs to combat social isolation, such as Befrienders or adult day services, are designed to stimulate social interactions.

Cultural Context

Occupational therapy evaluations include information gathered through interview about cultural influences on customs, beliefs, activity patterns, behavior standards, and expectations to design a culturally sensitive intervention (AOTA, 2008b). Caregiving is considered a cultural activity, with caregiving outcomes and experiences differing for ethnic groups (Dilworth-Anderson, Williams, & Gibson, 2002). Although the proportion of minority households providing caregiving is equal to the proportion of all households providing caregiving (21%; National Alliance for Caregiving, 2004), rates of institutionalization and use of formal caregiving services are lower in minority groups. Culturally defined roles can affect the selection of goals for evaluation and intervention. For example, if the primary caregiver is a wife, she may be reluctant to guide her husband in meal preparation or folding laundry if this is not a routine that is culturally acceptable to the couple. Likewise, guiding a male caregiver in providing personal care to a female may not be an acceptable task in certain cultures. Preserving dignity includes creating culturally favorable environments on the basis of the client's background and preferences.

Personal Context

The *personal context* includes age, gender, educational level, socioeconomic level, marital status, and family composition and should be part of the information obtained in the occupational profile. Alzheimer's disease is an age-related disease in that the greater majority of people in the early to middle stages of the disease are in their later years. Younger onset (before age 65) poses a particular challenge because decisions regarding workforce involvement are emotional and affect self-worth. Programs to promote occupational engagement for people in their 40s and 50s adapted to the needs of an individual who is cognitively impaired are scarce. Gender differences exist with Alzheimer's in part because of the longer life expectancies for women (U.S. Bureau of the Census, 2005). A decade ago, the ratio of women to men receiving long-term care institutional services was 3:1 (Congressional Budget Office, 2004). Level of education may influence the point at which the disease is diagnosed. People with a higher educational levels may be able to mask symptoms or may not exhibit the severity of symptoms until they are further along in the disease. Married people are able to live in the community for a longer period of time because of spousal caregiving availability. Socioeconomic status may influence the amount of assistance or support a client can access, which affects management of the limitations. Fewer offspring lead to a higher risk of supportive residence or institutional placement (Aykan, 2003).

Temporal Context

The *temporal context* refers to the "experience of time as shaped by engagement in occupations" (AOTA, 2008b, p. 645). Information about circadian rhythms (a measure of core body temperature and motor activity) is part of the initial interview in an occupational therapy evaluation because of the prevalence of "sundowner's syndrome" in people with Alzheimer's disease (Volicer, Harper, Manning, Goldstein, & Satlin, 2001). *Sundowners* is a common term referring to increased motor activity or agitation in the late afternoon or early evening hours. Altered sleep–wake cycles occur in the middle stages of the disease (Alzheimer's Association, 2008). Altered sleep–wake cycles occur when daytime becomes confused with nighttime. It is not unusual in the middle stages of the disease for the person with Alzheimer's disease to get up in the middle of the night and begin the day. When sleep–wake cycles are disturbed, the person with Alzheimer's disease may sleep most of the day. This situation is especially stressful for the primary caregiver who may experience sleep deprivation. Keeping a consistent routine with many daytime activities can stimulate the person to stay awake during the day and sleep better at night.

Virtual (Technology for Home Monitoring) Context

The *virtual context,* defined as a simulated environment that uses communication technologies in the absence of a human presence, can keep a person safe within his or her own home or in a residential facility. An interview can focus on information about behavioral issues related to wandering or exiting safe areas or potentially hazardous activities that require monitoring. High-tech assistive technologies include smart refrigerators that indicate by means of computer when food items need replenishing. They also include infra-red lights that indicate the presence of a person in a room or if a person has fallen. Smart TVs let a person know the stove has been left on or someone is at the door. Medication management systems use an alarm for pill distribution, but these have limited use in the middle and later stages of the disease. From global positioning devices in shoes, to motion detectors to monitor exiting behaviors, to electric appliances with safety shut-off mechanisms, new technologies can aid in promoting independence in the early to middle stages of the disease. In the middle stages of the disease, residential facilities use technology to restrict mobility and alert staff of nighttime waking. Low-tech assistive technologies can be of value, such as the Alzheimer's Association Safe Return program (Alzheimer's Association, 2008), a national tracking system for cognitively vulnerable adults. With any technology, consider the costs and feasibility of these technologies over the progression of the disease before making a recommendation to a client.

Activity Demands

Occupational therapy evaluation with people with Alzheimer's disease entails an exploration of the activity demands relative to the client's capabilities. This exploration frequently means interviewing the family members or primary caregivers in daily activity expectations and conducting an activity analysis. *Activity analysis* is breaking down the activity into components or steps of the process. The client may be competent to complete a task that is broken into step-by-step instructions or may be able to participate in portions of a task. The evaluation process should guide the practitioner in determining an educational plan for the caregiver. This plan may include the amount of assistance for each task, type of assistance, and safest method to approach the task.

In the early stages of Alzheimer's disease, complex tasks may present with difficulty, whereas simple tasks are generally successful. For instance, a client may be able to write checks to pay bills, but preparing and mailing the payment requires monitoring. Although multistep tasks are challenging, simple tasks are completed with success. A person may be able to complete one-step tasks but may become confused when two or three instructions are given in succession. For example, a client may be confused and frustrated by following a recipe with many ingredients and multiple steps, but he or she may be able to heat up a prepared meal in a microwave oven. Abstract instructions may be confusing, whereas concrete directions are followed with ease. An instruction such as "Get ready for dinner" is abstract, whereas "Put the plates on the table" is specific. The sequencing and timing of tasks can be barriers to participation. A person may be more alert earlier in the day and experience greater confusion in late afternoon. Space with heightened sensory stimulation may confuse an individual; multiple sources of sound, such as intercoms or radios, may be distracting and agitating. For example, the family may adapt the space by choosing a quiet, local restaurant rather than a bustling sports bar for lunch to minimize noise distractions. With well-designed caregiver education and modeling by the occupational therapy practitioner, the caregiver may become adept at activity analysis, problem solving, and natural adaptation of the tasks for successful participation.

Objects can stimulate a client's behavior. Through careful observation of the client's approach to activities, the occupational therapy practitioner can determine the manner in which clients use objects. The client may draw from habitual behavior when offered an object and naturally move through the steps of the task. For instance, when a client is handed a spoon, he or she may automatically begin to eat. These objects are prompts to initiate desired behavioral responses that can be a strategy to encourage occupational engagement.

Client Factors

Each client with Alzheimer's disease is a unique individual with a distinct set of underlying factors, both physical and motivational. The purpose of the evaluation is to determine what potential the client brings to the intervention process and to identify the barriers to optimal performance on the basis of physiological functions of body systems or personal values and beliefs. The assessments that correspond to specific body functions and are part of the domain of occupational practice can be used with this population with a caveat; if cognition alters the results of the assessment, another means of measuring that function needs to be selected. The individual may have visual deficits that impede unsupervised community mobility, but visual tests may require a cognitive–verbal response. The person with Alzheimer's may have apraxia that contributes to an unsafe environment but may not have the cognitive ability to learn to use a mobility support. A strong belief in self-determination may influence the desire to remain independent, but poor judgment because of cognitive decline may create an unsafe situation for living alone. In addition, evaluating the person's desire to pursue engagement in spiritual activities may influence recommendations in the intervention planning process. Spirituality is a component of quality of life and is connected to the dignity of each person regardless of cognitive awareness. For many areas of evaluation, the information is obtained through the clinical reasoning skills of a trained professional to identify which client factors justify intervention.

Intervention

Impact of Dementia

Dementia is a growing concern for health care professionals, with the prevalence estimated at 3.4 million

people in the United States alone; 2.4 million of that total is caused by Alzheimer's disease (Plassman et al., 2007). Beyond the emotional toll on people with the disease and family caregivers, the cost of care for Alzheimer's disease and other dementias ranked at the top of all conditions or diseases for Medicare beneficiaries in the 65 and older age group (Alzheimer's Association, 2009a). The major cost associated with Alzheimer's disease is for long-term care in the later stages of the disease. Pharmacological intervention for Alzheimer's disease has been found effective in slowing the progression of the disease for approximately 6 to 12 months, and active medical management has been proven effective in improving quality of life for people with the disease (Alzheimer's Association, 2009a). Active management refers to ongoing medical monitoring, treating coexisting conditions, and using supportive services for clients and caregivers, such as adult day services, caregiver education, and support groups. Over the course of the disease, the model of health care service delivery shifts from providing care in the natural environment, in the home and community, within a family-centered care model to supportive care in a facility within a medical or social services model.

Goals for Occupational Therapy Practice

For clients with Alzheimer's disease, the goal of occupational therapy intervention is to maximize the quality of life. According to the *Occupational Therapy Practice Framework* (AOTA, 2008b), *quality of life* is defined as engagement in occupation related to health and participation measured by involvement in work or volunteer activities, leisure, and daily living skills. The emphasis on quality of life is for both the client and caregiver and may involve identifying appropriate supports and resources to ensure safety and well-being. The progressive nature of the disease means occupational therapy intervention occurs at intervals over time. The goals of stage-based intervention change based on the needs of the client at each stage of the disease (Levy & Burns, 2005; see Boxes 2–5 for case studies in early, middle, and late stages of Alzheimer's disease). Intervention may entail therapeutic use of self by the occupational therapy practitioner to model a behavioral approach in working with a client, occupation-based therapeutic activities that have meaning for the client, consultation with the caregivers and other professionals working with the client regarding progress, family education about the disease progression, or advocacy for the client to receive community services (AOTA, 2008b). On a broader population-based scale, intervention may include developing programs for early to middle stages of the disease in community agencies; working on public policy for access to services; or administering services on an organizational, county, or state level.

With all interventions, the challenge is balancing client safety in performance with maximum independence. This balance may involve risk management— allowing greater independence per client choice at the risk of potential harm. The occupational therapy recommendation may be to encourage participation with strategies for safe performance or to limit participation because of the potential for injury and need to ensure safety. With that information, the client and family can make an informed decision with full knowledge of the risks and uncertainties.

Theory-Based Intervention

No single theoretical model guides occupational therapy intervention with people with Alzheimer's disease. The Allen Cognitive disabilities theory fits the stage-based model for intervention (Allen, Earhart, & Blue, 1992). This theory, developed initially for adults with schizophrenia and adapted for adults with dementia, guides the therapist to explain and predict occupational performance throughout the course of the disease. The ecological theoretical models— Person–Environment–Occupation (Law et al., 1996); Person–Environment–Occupation–Performance (Christiansen, Baum, & Bass-Haugen, 2005); and Ecology of Human Performance (Dunn, Brown, & Youngstrom, 2003)—emphasize the importance

of complex contextual factors, person factors, and occupational (or task) demands interacting with and influencing occupational performance (Brown, 2009). These theories inform the intervention planning by guiding the therapist to emphasize the role of the environment in creating a "just-right fit" with remaining cognitive abilities.

Occupational Adaptation theory highlights the naturally occurring adaptive responses a family makes to perpetuate the occupational performance of the family member (Schultz, 2009). This theory highlights the innate desire of the person to meet occupational challenges in the face of declining function. This theory guides the therapist to adapt the tasks to meet changing expectations for efficiency, effectiveness, and satisfaction with task performance.

The Model of Human Occupation (MOHO) emphasizes that human behavior is an outcome of volition, habituation, and performance capacity and is dynamic and context dependent (Kielhofner, 2008). According to MOHO, occupations contribute to and affect a person's self-organization, meaning that people become what they do. This model emphasizes the need for internal motivation to pursue occupations and occupational choices influenced by interests, emotions, values, habits, roles, and environments.

Family-Centered Care Model

A standard for occupational therapy intervention planning is to design interventions using a client-centered care model. This approach is a collaborative model with the therapist and client for selecting goals and developing a plan of care (Law, 1998). For the client with Alzheimer's disease who is dependent on a family caregiver, intervention planning is frequently conducted using a family-centered care model (Schaber, 2002). This model affects all steps of the evaluation and intervention planning process by including family caregivers in (1) obtaining information for the occupational history, (2) setting goals, and (3) exploring strengths and limitations. Another difference in a family-centered care model is that evidence for practice is drawn from occupational therapy and informed by social sciences research. Moreover, family members may be included in the intervention plan if they assist with self-care, productive activities, leisure pursuits, or social participation. Family-centered care is a collaboration with the therapist, client, and family member(s), and intervention is characterized by caregiver involvement through program implementation, education, and training. In the later stages of the disease, with a residential change to a memory care facility or long-term care institution, a team-centered care model is used to collaboratively select goals and develop a plan of care. At that point, the family becomes an integral part of the health care team.

Intervention Process

The occupational therapy process for intervention with people with Alzheimer's disease includes development of an intervention plan, implementation of the intervention plan, and intervention review (AOTA, 2008b). The plan, developed by an occupational therapist and corroborated with the

client (family), reflects client and caregiver needs, occupational therapy evaluation, knowledge of theory, and evidence guiding best practice. Intervention implementation is carried out by the occupational therapy practitioner and includes actions taken and activities selected that affect client performance or family responses. Throughout the intervention implementation, the client and family response is monitored and recorded, and the intervention is modified on the basis of progress toward the goals. The implementation review is a review of the plan and includes a periodic measure of progress toward the targeted outcomes (AOTA, 2008b).

Occupational Therapy Practice Framework and Alzheimer's Disease

The *Occupational Therapy Practice Framework* provides a rubric for occupational therapy intervention approaches (AOTA, 2008b; see Table 8). Interventions for people with Alzheimer's disease can be designed around creating, restoring, maintaining, modifying, or

Table 8. Occupational Therapy Intervention Approaches for People With Alzheimer's Disease and Family Caregivers, by Stage of Disease

Intervention Approach	Stage of Disease		
	Early	Middle	Late
Create or promote	Create opportunities to enhance daily involvement in community activities	Promote involvement through specialized memory loss programs	Involve client in adapted activities designed for changing abilities
Establish or restore	Restore functional independence using client and caregiver training and assistive technologies	Provide training in daily living skills, establishing consistency in performance patterns	Provide habituation training for communication systems and basic feeding, grooming, and dressing
Maintain	Build on past skills and habits to maintain present function	Develop functional maintenance programs for optimal engagement	Maintain physical, social, and occupational engagement at the optimal level
Modify	Adjust occupational demands, and increase environmental supports	Simplify daily tasks, modify cues, break down sequence to ability level	Guide with external supports to enhance participation in portions of the task
Prevent	Provide prevention education in targeted areas (e.g., falls, geographic orientation, medication management, financial oversight, options for community mobility)	Encourage activity engagement by initiating task and offering step-by-step guidance to minimize daytime sleep	Stimulate activity in physical, social, and functional areas through sensory inputs

preventing deterioration of occupational performance. Interventions that create or promote occupational performance provide opportunities to entice participation using the client's abilities and skills, such as adult day service programs or specialized activity programs for people with memory loss.

Restorative interventions are designed for people in the early stages of the disease, when the capacity for new learning exists. These interventions may include training in alternative methods for community mobility or new systems for communication such as pre-programmed telephones. An example of *maintenance* interventions may be the use of personnel to guide the client in occupational performance offering assistance for select portions of the task that are beyond the client's ability level. These interventions may include increasing consistency in schedules, task methods, approaches, routines, and daily caregivers. Interventions to *modify* the activity demands include compensatory approaches to daily activities. This approach is primarily in the form of environmental adaptation, activity analysis to simplify task performance demands, and caregiver training to guide the performance using appropriate cues. *Prevention* interventions are designed to ensure safety in occupational performance and to counteract occupational deprivation. The individualized intervention for each client requires the expertise and clinical reasoning skills of the occupational therapy practitioner. Interventions target areas of occupation (work or volunteer, IADLs, ADLs, leisure, social participation, sleep/rest), performance skills (motor and praxis, sensory–perceptual, emotional regulation, cognitive, communication and social skills) and patterns (habits, routines, roles, rituals), activity demands (objects, space and social demands, sequencing/timing, required actions and body functions/structures), client factors (body functions and body structures, values, beliefs, and spirituality), and contexts and environments (cultural, personal, temporal, virtual, physical, social; AOTA, 2008b).

Discontinuation of Service

Discontinuation of occupational therapy intervention services occurs when clients meet their goals or appear to have reached their maximum potential in the targeted outcomes. With psychoeducational services or caregiver training programs, discontinuation of service occurs when the caregiver demonstrates an understanding of the program and can implement the functional maintenance program competently. Services also may be discontinued if the client refuses intervention or if the family, as legal guardian, requests an end to therapy. Measures of progress are taken at the time of discharge and documented in the appropriate medical or agency record. Outcomes may measure a change in occupational performance, such as greater effectiveness or efficiency, adaptations to compensate for cognitive declines, measures of health or wellness based on medical or family report, increased participation, prevention of excess disability or an absence of decline, or perceived improvement in quality of life of the client or caregiver (AOTA, 2008b). A follow-up may be scheduled to inquire about progress and maintenance of goals. With Alzheimer's disease, the follow-up may range from 6 months to 1 year because of the slow progression of the disease. Occupational therapy can reactivate when a referral is generated based on a change of condition or rapid decline in level of performance.

Documentation

An essential part of the evaluation and intervention process is documentation (AOTA, 2008a). This includes a documented evaluation report with a summary of occupational performance (see Box 1. Sample Evaluation Report) intervention plan with measurable goals, progress notes with dates of service, and discontinuation summary with recommendations and/or referrals. Generally, for an occupational therapy intervention to be considered covered under the Medicare program, a service must be

- Prescribed by a physician and furnished according to a written plan of care, established by the therapist and approved by the physician
- Performed by a qualified occupational therapist or by an occupational therapy assistant under the supervision of an occupational therapist
- Reasonable and necessary for the treatment of the person's illness or injury (Centers for Medicare and Medicard Services, 2008).

Although a mental health diagnosis does not preclude Medicare coverage of occupational therapy, the program does require that goals be related to the patient's condition, reasonable, and measurable. Therefore, it is very important that occupational therapy documentation reflect valid anticipated outcomes of treatment based on a supportable clinical assessment of the individual's condition.

Categorizing Intervention for People With Alzheimer's Disease

Interventions for people with Alzheimer's disease can be categorized in different ways, for instance, by stage of the disease (early, middle, or late stage), by setting (home, assisted living, memory care, institutional care), by caregiver availability (spousal/continuous, adult offspring/periodic, paid aide/scheduled), and by client capabilities (high risk vs. low risk factors). The problem in categorizing intervention approaches is that there is broad individual variation in multiple areas throughout the course of the disease. A general impression of client skills and capabilities can be gained through standardized testing at each stage of the disease; however, each client has a unique constellation of symptoms, degrees of motor and language involvement, behavioral issues, and caregiver availability. These differences require tailoring interventions or individualizing care. For example, one intervention approach is training in memory aides. Some people in the early stages may benefit from training in memory aides for medication management, whereas others experience increased confusion using a medication box and frequently make errors in self-administration. Another intervention is the use

of signage. A person in the middle stage in a memory care facility may be able to follow signage for reminders to locate their room, whereas another may disregard or misinterpret the visual cues. Because there are many factors to be considered with each unique person with the disease, best practice for occupational therapy intervention is tailored to the individual and family/caregiver.

Intervention Areas of Occupation

Interventions in areas of occupation predominantly focus on caregiver education using environmental or compensatory strategies (Graff et al., 2006). An occupational therapy educational intervention should be tailored specifically to the person and family seeking services. The goal is maximum participation in areas of occupation at the desired level of the client, weighing risks for safety versus autonomy. Alzheimer's disease is predominantly found in populations ages 65 or older, although younger onset does appear with people in their 50s and early 60s. Therefore, the areas of occupation affected are those in which older adults are engaged, primarily work or volunteer, IADLs, ADLs, leisure, social participation, and sleep. In general, occupational performance goals in the early stage are directed toward participation in work or IADLs; in the middle stage, leisure, social participation, and ADLs; and in the later stages of the disease, social participation and basic ADLs (see Table 9).

Work or Volunteer Activities

Concerns about performance in work or volunteer responsibilities are one of the first indicators of cognitive involvement. In younger-onset Alzheimer's disease, care planning focuses on maintenance of valued occupations (Bentham & LaFontaine, 2005). In many cases, the job has been gradually adapted as tasks that prove frustrating are substituted with less challenging work. A critical decision for the client is when to leave paid employment or withdraw from a volunteer position. At any age, this decision has a

Table 9. Occupational Therapy Intervention for Early, Middle, and Late Stages of Alzheimer's Disease

Stage of Disease	Areas of Occupation	Occupational Therapy Intervention
Early stage	Work/volunteer IADLs Leisure Social participation	Create opportunities to engage in work/volunteer tasks adapted to client capacity Modify environmental and activity demands to reduce frustration and provide caregiver education and training in modifications Maintain safe engagement in IADLs with appropriate supports and resources Establish primary and secondary social network with family and community Promote involvement in leisure activities of choice; adapt leisure activities to client capacity
Middle stage	ADLs Leisure Social participation Sleep	Maximize engagement in ADLs through compensatory and environmental adaptations Train caregivers in tailored activity programs Create opportunities for leisure skills identifying adequate supervision and concerns for safety Pursue community-based programs designed for people with cognitive loss Prevent sleep disturbances through active engagement in daytime activities
Late stage	ADLs Social participation Sleep	Maintain client factors to participate in ADLs with caregiver support and training Modify approach to social participation to meet the need for human contact Prevent co-morbidities related to decreased movement during sleep/rest

Note. ADLs = activities of daily living; IADLs = instrumental activities of daily living.

major impact on self-esteem, occupational engagement, and financial dependability, but it is especially distressing to the 50-year-old client in the generative period of his or her life span. The occupational therapist can conduct an activity analysis to determine which tasks may be adapted and which should be discontinued to ensure safe and productive work.

IADLs

In the early stages of the disease, the focus of intervention is on safe IADL performance with driving, meal preparation, home maintenance (e.g., lawn care, snow removal, home exterior care) and homemaking (e.g., cleaning, shopping, repairs, laundry), medication and health management (e.g., scheduling appointments), and personal finance (e.g., banking, balancing checkbook, paying bills). A critical concern is when to discontinue driving. Although some people relinquish driving when they feel unsafe or experience getting lost, others resist driving cessation into the middle stages of the disease. Multiple factors need to be considered before making a recommenda-

tion to give up the car keys. A formal referral for a driving evaluation can support the family in making an informed decision.

The occupational therapy practitioner can modify or compensate for activities in IADL performance in meal preparation, medication management, financial management, and home maintenance through activity analysis or can alter the client responsibilities for success. Likewise, occupational therapy practitioners can provide information about transportation options to allow persons with Alzheimer's disease to participate in their valued occupations outside the home and within the community. Caregiver education and training is a key intervention strategy to promote participation and engagement in day-to-day activities.

ADLs

The areas of ADLs affected generally surface in the middle stage of the disease and include dressing (e.g., selecting clothing, donning and doffing, managing laundry), grooming, showering/bathing (e.g., behavioral resistance), and eating. At the stage that ADLs are performed inconsistently or inadequately, the goal of intervention is to balance the amount and type of assistance with the capabilities of the client. This assistance entails adaptations to the activity, training of caregivers, or compensatory interventions. An adaptation may be to reduce the articles of clothing in a closet to shirts and pants that coordinate (vs. clash) to encourage independent selection of clothing. People may forget to eat or drink fluids during the day, precipitating agitation or sensory seeking to satisfy their needs. On the contrary, they may forget they have eaten and will appear insatiable (Fagan, 2002). They may have a clear preference for certain types of food, leading to imbalanced nutritional intake. Offering fluids periodically during the day and monitoring daily nutrition is important at this stage. Altering the approach to showering or bathing, such as towel baths, may reduce resistance for the caregiver and maintain proper hygiene in the middle to later stages of the disease.

Leisure

Leisure and social participation become challenging as the need for supervision increases and interaction skills diminish. Leisure activities may require gradual and continual adaptations and re-adaptations as the disease progresses. Promoting leisure skills includes modifying the activity for continued engagement or adding supervision to the activity. For example, a person who enjoys biking may need a companion to prevent getting lost or ride tandem with a bike partner. In middle to later stages of the disease with increasing motor involvement, a tricycle may be needed to replace the bicycle along with a designated bike path route. Biking is an example of a repetitive, gross motor, one-step, familiar activity that can be encouraged to maintain engagement in leisure activity over time (Levy, 1986).

Physical activity is an important part of leisure related to health and well-being. Home-based exercise programs that included aerobic activity, strength training, balance, and flexibility training were found to improve physical function and mobility in people with Alzheimer's disease (Teri et al., 2003). Studies support engagement in physical activity throughout the course of the disease, including for institutionalized people with dementia. Lazowski and colleagues (1999) found benefits with aerobic training on cognitive performance with nursing home residents. Benefits also include improving overall strength and coordination to reduce the risk for falls and injury.

Social Participation

A person's social circle gradually diminishes as symptoms of the disease become more apparent. It is not uncommon to observe withdrawal from clubs and civic or community groups, church groups, and even family events by the middle stages of the disease. For some people, their retirement period was organized by their social activities, and retreating from social involvement leaves them occupationally disengaged. The stigma surrounding Alzheimer's disease, along with a tendency for people to withdraw socially, is a barrier to discussing the challenges a person encounters. Some, albeit limited, organized community activities promote and support involvement in the early stages of the disease; adult day service programs structure social involvement in the later stages of the disease.

Sleep

Sleep cycles are disrupted in 25% of clients with Alzheimer's disease (Bliwise, 2004). Interventions may include increasing leisure activities such as exercise or hobbies that limit excessive daytime napping. Other standard sleep promotion measures can be suggested, such as limiting caffeinated beverages, encouraging consistent routines before bedtime, turning off the television before sleeping, and instituting approaches to calm the person during the night (American Academy Family Physicians, 2008).

Box 1. Sample Evaluation Report

OCCUPATIONAL THERAPY COGNITIVE PERFORMANCE EVALUATION

Memory Clinic Report

Client: Tina Bellows MR# 002349087 DOB 9/7/1933

Date of Order: 5/6/06

Date of Service: 5/9/06 Time: 2:00 p.m. to 3:15 p.m., 75 min

Referring Physician: Dr. H. Turnquist

Date of onset: 4/24/06

Diagnosis: Alzheimer's disease

Prognosis: Increased supervision and assistance will be needed in IADLs and ADLs as condition progresses

Problem: Moderate memory problems

Functional History:

Client is married and has three children. She attended the occupational therapy evaluation with her spouse, George, her son, Evan, and two daughters, Theresa and Lois. Her husband is the primary caregiver. She has a high school education. She is 77 years old and European American.

The major problem reported is memory. Client's perception of memory/thinking difficulties are "Well, I know all my kids' and grandkids' names."

Family members' perception of memory-thinking difficulties are as follows: "The biggest problem is we can talk about something and the next minute she forgets; it's short-term memory."

At this point, there are no safety concerns that would warrant a change in residence.

- Client lives with her husband in a single-family home. They live on a farm, and her son, Evan, lives next door. There are family members and workers on the farm at all hours. Tina spends most of her time in the house engaged in homemaking activities.
- Home maintenance activities (shoveling snow, mowing lawn, raking, window washing, repairs): She is active mowing the lawn with a riding lawn mower and completes most of the yardwork and simple repairs. She has a large garden that she tends for a portion of the year.
- Home management (laundry, cleaning, grocery shopping, bed making, vacuuming): She manages the home independently, including laundry, cleaning, vacuuming. Her husband partners with her to do the weekly shopping; she uses grocery lists. She has a hired cleaning person to complete heavy cleaning weekly.
- Driving: Tina drives on the farm property and 2 miles on a rural road to church. She does not drive beyond a few miles, and the roads are sparsely traveled and familiar.
- Medication management (simple or complex [> 4 pills] medication regime): She has a complex medication schedule, and her daughter sets up her pills weekly in a medication management system. She takes them with no reminders.
- Personal finances (bill paying and banking): Tina does most of the personal finances, but her son, Evan, makes out the farmhand payroll, and Tina writes the checks. Evan checks and balances the finances weekly.
- Meal preparation: Tina is responsible for cooking the noon meal for those who work on the farm. This meal could be for up to 5 or 6 people. She independently makes a complex meal (meat, potatoes, vegetable, salad, dessert) and reports no errors in meal prep, although her family members report she is tense and irritable around meal service.

(continued)

Box 1. Sample Evaluation Report *(cont.)*

- ADLs (dressing, grooming, toileting, bathing): She is independent in dressing, grooming, showering.
- Leisure activities: She and her husband eat out nightly because she cooks a full meal at lunchtime. She is active in her church, the Red Hat Society, and occasionally goes to the casino with her husband. She used to have a larger social circle, but this circle is diminishing. Most of her leisure time is currently shared with her husband.
- Summary of occupational participation: Tina is occupationally engaged, spending most of her day home-making and cooking for the farmworkers. She has reduced her social activities outside of her immediate family and spends non–work time with her husband. Her family members have expressed concerns about her ability to continue meal preparation and have offered to hire additional help. They are very supportive and willing to monitor, supervise, and assist with IADL activities.

Score: Cognitive Performance Test (CPT) (Burns, 2006)
Subtask Scores:
Medbox 4.5/6
Shop 4.5/6
Dress 5.0/5
Travel 5.0/6
Wash 5.0/5
Phone 4.5/6
Toast 4.0/5
Total CPT 32.5/39 or 4.6/5.6

Test Narrative:
Medbox: Tina was able to get Fluida correct but had errors on the other three measures and was unable to correct with specific cues.
Shop: She chose a belt that did not fit and needed a verbal cue to look at bottom belts.
Dress: No errors on task.
Travel: She followed mostly visual cues rather than the map and passed her destination; she asked questions rather than pointing out her destination.
Wash: No errors on task.
Phone: Located phone number; dialed three times; asked the wrong question.
Toast: Tina required a repeat of verbal directions after the toast popped up.

Cognitive Performance Test Interpretation (adapted from Burns, 1991, 1996):
Tina appears to function close to Level 4.6 behaviors. She shows impairments in memory, judgment, reasoning, and planning ahead. People at this level have significant difficulty with activities that rely on abstract thought processes, such as reading, writing, and calculating. She is able to perform overlearned activities, drawing from long-term procedural memory, but may have difficulty learning new skills or procedures. She seems to be able to self-correct task errors with specific cues but frequently is not aware of the error until it is pointed out. Complex daily tasks appear to elicit anxiety. At this level, hazardous activities may need to be monitored for safe performance or restricted to ensure safety. Tina appears to have minimal awareness of her cognitive limitations. She is able to make use of long-time coping measures to continue to manage most ADLs and does perform familiar activities, the most challenging being preparing a complex meal for multiple people daily. At present, she appears to be occupationally engaged, due to a supportive fam-

Box 1. Sample Evaluation Report *(cont.)*

ily that is willing to adapt her daily activities, and she is actively engaged in farm life where she is comfortable and tasks are familiar. She has limited social activity outside of her family and the farm. She does engage in church groups.

Mobility and Physical Function:
Normal gait and upper extremity movement patterns.

Summary of Findings:
Tina appears to need supervision in complex IADL activities and is able to complete her ADLs independently. Driving ability is questionable at this level, especially considering her confusion around directions. Medications need to be monitored, along with handling personal finances and farm finances. Hazardous tasks such as the use of the stove and any farm machinery should be closely supervised. She needs supervision in unfamiliar environments because of the possibility of her getting lost. She does not seem receptive to assistance with the farm tasks, especially preparing meals and cleaning, and she does not want to relinquish her independence.

Intervention Goal:
Client and family will verbalize understanding of cognitive evaluation results and implications for safety, medication management, finances, driving, meal prep, shopping, and social isolation.

Intervention and Education Completed:
Discussed and interpreted evaluation results, CPT score of 4.6/5.6, and implications for performance of IADLs and work and leisure pursuits with Tina and her family. Strategies for engaging in meal prep activities, monitoring medications, sharing financial management tasks with son, and caution around driving/community mobility were discussed. Education was provided in the areas of (1) home safety; (2) supervision with medications, finances, meals, and homemaking tasks; (3) caution around driving beyond farm and church areas because of the potential for getting lost; and (4) poor insight or lack of awareness of judgment and problem-solving impairments. Family caregiving materials were provided for Level 4.5.

Client/Family Response:
The client and family seemed favorable about the recommendations regarding seeking additional supports in the farm tasks with those tasks where there is visible evidence of frustration. Tina was resistant to making any changes in her daily routine and feels confident that she can handle driving and managing IADLs with no assistance. A family meeting will follow this evaluation.

Addendum:
A family meeting was held after the occupational therapy evaluation. Dr. H. Turnquist facilitated the meeting with the family; the family caregiving center counselors also were present. The occupational therapist reviewed the results of the CPT and implications for additional supports in IADL activities. The family was cautioned about Tina's driving beyond a 2-mile radius and the need for supervision in driving in unfamiliar areas. The Memory Clinic team recommended a formal driving evaluation if the family needed additional support to plan for cessation of driving in the future. The family was encouraged to support Tina's social engagement and continuation of those tasks where she can complete a portion of the activity with assistance and monitoring for the portion that is beyond her capabilities. Her daughter will set up medications and monitor for errors in self-administration. Her son will continue to assist with finances, allowing her to continue with check writing. Her husband and daughter will monitor frustration levels with meal prep and household management. They will seek a paid assistant to help with meal prep and with gradually increasing home management tasks as the need arises. Dr. Turnquist answered numerous questions about the diagnosis and medications, and the family caregiving center counselors provided resource information for future planning and support.

Box 2. Case Study—Mild Cognitive Decline, Early-Stage Alzheimer's Disease

Occupational Profile

Verna Caldwell is a 78-year-old, retired widow who lives independently in a single-family home in a metropolitan area. She has three children. Her son Ted and daughter Frida live close by, and a daughter, Ann, lives 3 hours away. She reports that her memory problems are not a constant thing and that the more water she drinks, the better her memory becomes. She hires someone to complete home maintenance activities, including mowing the lawn and washing windows outdoors. She takes care of all home management, including laundry, cleaning, bed making, and vacuuming, and she has a cleaning woman come every other week. She is able to grocery shop for a few items, but her daughter goes with her on weekends to plan meals for the week. She drives independently in familiar areas and occasionally drives to see her daughter 3 hours away. Aside from this long-distance trip, she restricts herself to local streets with no freeway driving or driving at night. She has had one minor fender scrape. She takes no medications except for an inhaler PRN. She handles all personal finances and reported that this is an important activity to maintain. She reports no errors in paying bills or overdrafts. She reports ability to prepare a light meal independently, although she eats out three times a week and eats frequently with her children. She is independent in ADLs (dressing, grooming, toileting, bathing).

Verna enjoyed golf and bridge, and she formerly had an active social life with a group of friends from her church and senior community center, but she seems to be withdrawing from these activities. She has two dogs and used to walk them daily for exercise but reports being too busy to continue this activity. She stated she has a fear of falling because the dogs are eager to move quickly. She has a very engaged family and is actively involved with her four grandchildren.

Her family members report that they are comfortable with Verna's independent living situation but reported some concerns about her driving distances, her nutritional status, her decreasing level of physical and social activity, and fears concerning her ability to manage her finances. They recently found some unpaid bills. They reported that she occasionally will forget an appointment, or they need to remind her of the appointment in the morning to make sure she is ready and available.

Analysis of Occupational Performance

Verna scored 26 on the Mini-Mental Status Exam (Folstein, Folstein, & McHugh, 1975) and a 1.0 on the Clinical Dementia Rating scale (Morris, 1993; 0.5 is *questionable dementia*, 1.0 is *mild*, 2.0 is *moderate*, and 3.0 is *severe*) and was referred to occupational therapy. She was administered the Kitchen Task Assessment (Baum & Edwards, 1993) and received a summed score of 5.0, which corresponds to a mild stage of dementia (range, 0 = *independent*, 18 = *not capable on 6 task components*). She required verbal cues to initiate, organize, and complete the task and physical assistance for judgment and safety. A mild or early stage is often indicative of a change in memory, judgment, and reasoning abilities. In the early stage, complex tasks such as calculated finances, using a map for driving directions, making a complicated recipe, or managing a complex medication schedule begin to show difficulties. There may be limitations in self-awareness of disability; the person is generally not aware of an error until it is pointed out and with effort is able to self-correct. In the early stage, the ability to make financial or residential decisions is difficult without family support. Leisure activities continue but diminish in frequency, and the person relies on family and friends to plan and carry out activities.

Intervention Plan

Occupational therapy intervention goals:

- Client and family members will verbalize an understanding of cognitive evaluation results and implications for safety precautions, specifically driving in unfamiliar areas, carrying identification, and accessing emergency services.
- Client and family members will receive 7 weeks of home-based occupational therapy to improve performance in daily activities (Graff et al., 2003, 2007).
- Client and family members will identify methods to monitor finances, such as online access to accounts by a person designated with power of attorney, setting up automatic bill pay, and monthly monitoring of bills and payments (Kolanowski, 2001).

Box 2. Case Study—Mild Cognitive Decline, Early-Stage Alzheimer's Disease *(cont.)*

- Client and family members will comprehend the need for continued physical activity and strengthening for falls prevention (Jensen, Nyberg, Gustafson & Lundin-Olsson, 2003; Toulotte, Fabre, Dangremont, Lensel, & Thevenon, 2003) and will identify alternative strategies for community mobility if and when driving ceases (Passini, Rainville, Marchand, & Joanette, 1998).
- Family members will monitor meals by increasing weekly shared meals, providing heat-and-serve meals with clear, large-print instructions on microwave oven, and checking periodically for weight loss or indicators of poor nutrition (Graff et al., 2006).

Box 3. Case Study—Moderate Cognitive Decline, Middle-Stage Alzheimer's Disease

Occupational Profile

Florence Coffman is a 79-year-old widow who currently lives with her daughter Sally for a portion of the year and her son Fred for part of the year. She sold the family home 3 years ago and has been residing with her children ever since. She reports moderate memory problems but is content with the living arrangement and is pleasant and articulate about her needs and desires. One desire is to live with family members rather than a supportive living environment. The family members' perception of memory thinking difficulties are that Florence has poor short-term recall and limited judgment, which affects her ability to be safely home alone during the day. She does participate in some IADLs; she has no home maintenance or home management responsibilities, although, when guided by a family member, she does assist with portions of activities such as vacuuming, setup, and meal preparation (chopping vegetables for salads and setting the table with verbal cues) folding towels, and cleaning her bedroom (making the bed). She assists with grocery shopping when paired with a family member. She voluntarily relinquished driving 3 years ago when she moved from her home. She has medications set up, and she self-administers with reminders. Her children handle all personal finances, but she is able to purchase using a debit card and sign checks for paying bills. She is beginning to show a need for monitoring for ADLs (dressing, grooming, showering) for consistency and competent performance. She has an aversion to bathing and becomes agitated before the task. She used to be an avid knitter (at present she is able to knit squares with some errors) and enjoys crafts. She completes simple crossword puzzles, reads the headlines of the newspaper, and walks supervised in the neighborhood. Because of the change in residence, she is not active socially outside of her family. Florence did express that she is happy with her children and that she took care of her mother before she died.

Florence's daughter and son expressed concerns about her time alone during the day. They believe she needs more supervision than they are able to provide because they work, and she is home alone for up to 9 hours. Although she has not gotten lost, they expressed a need to more closely monitor her daytime activities and the potential for wandering beyond the neighborhood. She has not had an incident using the stove, but they asked her not to cook when she is home alone. She heats up a prepared lunch in the microwave.

Analysis of Occupational Performance

Florence scored a 19 on the MMSE (Folstein, Folstein, & McHugh, 1975) and was referred to occupational therapy. She was administered the Cognitive Performance Test (Burns, 2006) and received a 4.0. This score indicates a need for assistance with all IADLs and monitoring or supervision with ADLs, including dressing, grooming, and bathing. A person with this score may be able to perform ADLs, but performance is inconsistent or inefficient. Setting up and initiating a dressing task may improve independent performance but generally requires continual cueing and

(continued)

handing clothing items for completion. The person can eat independently with the meal presented and prompts at intervals. Showering may require physical assistance to reduce resistance, or alternative methods for personal hygiene, such as towel baths, may need to be explored. The person may become anxious when alone without verbal reassurance from a family member or caregiver. At this level, potential hazards need to be averted, such as use of the stove, electrical appliances, machinery, or self-administration of medications. Behavioral changes may require increased supervision. The person may withdraw socially and need specialized activities adapted to his or her ability level.

Intervention Plan

Occupational therapy intervention goals:

- Client and family will verbalize an understanding of the cognitive evaluation results and implications for safety precautions, specifically wandering beyond the home environment (Namazi & Johnson, 1992b), carrying identification, and accessing emergency telephone assistance (Topo, Jylha, & Laine, 2002).
- Client and family member will promote engagement in portions of homemaking activities and understand the need to initiate the task; guide performance; and guide the client with prompts, cues, and assistance (Dooley & Hinojosa, 2004).
- Client and family member will identify methods to promote independence in ADLs, specifically setting out clothing for dressing and supplies for grooming, adapting showering activity by creating a routine procedure with music to minimize agitation (Gotell, Brown, & Ekman, 2003), and providing reminders to complete oral care (Graff et al. 2006).
- Client and family member will explore options for adult day services and transportation to the day programs for a physical strengthening program (Jenson et al., 2004), family-style meals for social involvement (Altus, Engelman, & Mathews, 2002), and adapted art activities designed for people with dementia (Rentz, 2002).

Box 4. Case Study—Moderately Severe Cognitive Decline, Middle- to Late-Stage Alzheimer's Disease

Occupational Profile

Tilda Fromm is an 85-year-old widow who lives in a memory care residential facility. She has a son, Greg, and daughter, Lily, who live within 30 miles of the facility. Tilda was unable to respond to questions when asked to describe her memory and functional difficulties. She did respond to greetings and participated in informal conversation, offering comments using strong verbal abilities that did not match her functional abilities. In the supported living environment, Tilda has assistance with all IADLs and some ADLs. She feeds herself with meals presented and prompts to initiate the eating process; all meals are brought to her room. The family has concerns about her nutritional status, reporting she "takes a long time to eat" and does not have the encouragement she needs to maintain her weight. She has assistance with selecting clothing, and her family reports she is capable of donning articles of clothing when items are handed to her but often will accept dressing assistance. She has occasional incontinence during the day. She participates in limited activities outside her room and expressed concerns about finding her way back to her room. She uses a walker in her room and a wheelchair when she leaves the efficiency apartment to go to the common area or out of the building. The only activity she reported to enjoy was reading. Her former activity interests include gardening, cooking, walking, and hiking. She enjoys all types of reading—newspapers and books, including mystery novels. She reported to be able to comprehend what she read, but the family thought this notion was questionable.

Box 4. Case Study—Moderately Severe Cognitive Decline, Middle- to Late-Stage Alzheimer's Disease *(cont.)*

Tilda's daughter expressed concerns about the limited activity participation in the facility. Tilda is reluctant to leave her room and participate in group activities and only will attend when accompanied by her daughter. Her daughter is available to visit only on weekends because of a demanding work schedule. Tilda has limited social interaction during the day and refuses to eat meals in a common dining area.

Analysis of Occupational Performance

Tilda scored an 8 on the MMSE (Folstein, Folstein, & McHugh, 1975) and was referred to occupational therapy. She was administered the Cognitive Performance Test (Burns, 2006) and received a 3.3 total score. Her abstract thinking at this level is very impaired with an inability to reason, plan, problem solve, or remember. Objects in her environment stimulate and cue behaviors; for instance, a glass placed in front of her will stimulate drinking, a sweater handed to her will stimulate donning clothing. There is limited object permanence in that only objects in sight are considered. She has lack of focus in initiating an activity and may need cues and probes to stay attentive because of her distractibility. She is able to participate in portions of activity, especially those tasks that are overlearned. The quality of her performance requires monitoring. ADLs need to be supervised with prompts, cues, or demonstration to complete the tasks. Daily activities require 24-hour supervision in a safe environment.

Intervention Plan

Occupational therapy intervention goals:

- Client and family will verbalize an understanding of cognitive evaluation results and implications for safety precautions, specifically 24-hour supervision and assistance with all ADLs.
- Facility staff will promote engagement in facility activities designed for a dementia care unit to combat social isolation (Kovach & Stearns, 1994). Staff members will provide signage and environmental cues to facilitate her finding her room and reducing her anxiety about leaving her room (Gibson, MacLean, Borrie, & Geiger, 2004; Nolan, Mathews, & Harrison, 2001). Staff will be trained to carry out activities tailored to her interests and ability level (Kolanowski, 2001) and will encourage family-style meals in the dining room (Altus et al., 2002).
- Facility staff will include the client in portions of homemaking tasks such as making the bed and dusting her furniture (Dooley & Hinojosa, 2004).
- Facility staff will receive training to provide effective prompts, cues, and assistance for ADLs, specifically dressing, grooming, showering, and oral care (Rogers et al., 1999). She will be prompted to void on a scheduled timetable during the day (Skelly & Flint, 1995).

Box 5. Case Study—Severe Cognitive Decline, Late-Stage Alzheimer's Disease

Occupational Profile

Trudeau Boucher is a 78-year-old man. He was unable to respond to questions when asked to describe his memory and functional difficulties. He did respond to greetings and participated in informal conversation, offering comments that were off topic but animated responses. His wife, Arlene, was present during the interview and answered all of the questions regarding functional status. She reported that Trudeau lives with her in the upper duplex that they own. He is dependent in all IADLs, and she provides moderate assistance with all ADLs. He feeds himself independently with one item of food at a time and hand-over-hand assistance; he is able to dress himself when the clothes are provided and the task is initiated by Arlene. He is able to groom with task setup and verbal or physically initiated assistance. He

(continued)

Box 5. Case Study—Severe Cognitive Decline, Late-Stage Alzheimer's Disease *(cont.)*

is able to toilet when brought to the bathroom and the procedure is initiated. He requires physical assistance from one person with bathing. Trudeau participates in limited activities inside and outside the apartment. For the most part, he watches TV and sleeps frequently during the day. His wife reported she is able to leave him alone for up to 20 minutes if she is in the yard or on the grounds. Arlene reported that she used to try to involve him in portions of daily home-making tasks, but lately she does most tasks alone. She reported that he sleeps well through the night most of the time, but on occasion will experience a period of anxiety and has nighttime incontinence, which is managed with disposable undergarments. He has had two falls in the past year without injuries. He is compliant and is physically easy to guide. A neighbor is available to provide supervision if Arlene is off the premises, but Trudeau becomes anxious and does not like it when Arlene is gone. Trudeau was teary-eyed on and off throughout the occupational therapy evaluation.

Arlene expressed concerns about the increasing need to provide continual supervision and her inability to obtain respite services to go shopping or to visit her friends. She has concerns about guiding Trudeau up and down the apartment staircase alone. She observed that his activity levels are gradually receding, and she does not have interest in guiding his leisure time activities. If his nighttime sleep disruptions or episodes of incontinence increase, she may consider a residential placement in a memory care unit in a skilled nursing facility.

Analysis of Occupational Performance

Trudeau did not score on the MMSE (Folstein, Folstein, & McHugh, 1975) and was observed in occupational therapy participating in a dressing and eating activity. He handled objects but was not aware of their use; he was rated as severe cognitive–functional decline with progression from concrete to object-centered thought processes. At this stage, the person requires one-to-one assistance for task initiation and continual guidance. Task objects, when handed to the client, will get the task started, but the client does not independently carry through with the task. Rote activities, especially overlearned skills, can be stimulated with familiar objects, and the person will manipulate the object for short periods of time. The client may cooperate with portions of ADLs, such as removing a coat, when the activity is initiated and prompted or may resist with behavioral symptoms associated with the dementia; the person requires close, 24-hour supervision, and hazardous activities need to be restricted.

Intervention Plan

Occupational therapy intervention goals:

- Client and family will verbalize understanding of cognitive evaluation results and implications for the need for 24-hour supervision and restrictions around potentially hazardous activities. Family caregiver training will be provided for a falls prevention program (Savage & Matheis-Kraft, 2001) and sleep hygiene program (McCurry et al., 2003).
- Client and family members will promote engagement in portions of ADLs such as moving the shaver on the face when guided, donning a shirt with hand-over-hand assistance, feeding self finger foods, and washing self in a tub with guidance and assist (Rogers et al., 1999). Caregiver will be trained in timed voiding during day-time hours (Ostaszkiewicz, Johnston, & Roe, 2004b).
- Referral to social services for adult day services (Schacke & Zank, 2006) or residential memory care programs that provide some personal care services (showering) and adapted leisure activities (Buettner, 1999), specifically, a multisensory exercise program (Heyn, 2003).
- Referral to social services for respite care for the caregiver and local Alzheimer's support groups (Hepburn et al., 2005; Mittleman, Ferris, Shulman, Steinsberg, & Levin, 1996).

Evidence for Interventions in Areas of Occupation

Several studies have examined the areas of occupation in intervention for Alzheimer's type dementia. Graff and colleagues (2003), in a Level III pretest–posttest study, demonstrated the effectiveness of occupational therapy client-centered home visits for people with dementia in the mild to moderate stages of the disease. In the 7-week session spanning hospital (2 weeks) to home (5 weeks) intervention, they found that occupational performance improved in motor and process skills and caregiver competence. Graff and colleagues (2007), in a Level I randomized controlled trial, demonstrated effectiveness in community-based occupational therapy intervention for people with mild to moderate dementia. Additional findings from this research were published in 2006 and 2008. Their results indicated increased client function, caregiver sense of coherence, client and caregiver health status and mood, quality of life, and sense of control. The biweekly (10-session) intervention focused on environmental and compensatory strategies.

Limited success has been shown in interventions that incorporate direct training of the client in areas of occupation. Avila and colleagues (2004), in a Level III study, examined memory training in five participants with probable Alzheimer's in three IADL areas: phone use, diary use, and food preparation. The 14-week intervention showed a trend toward improvement, although the only area showing significant change was with a functional test measure. Training in phone use using photos and programmed numbers did not appear to affect phone usage for six community-dwelling residents with mild dementia in a Level IV descriptive case study (Topo et al., 2002). By contrast, Fitzsimmons and Buettner (2003), in a Level II study with a delayed intervention control group, found that a therapeutic cooking program for 5 days a week for 2 weeks significantly reduced agitation and decreased passivity. This study supported engaging people with dementia in functional activities for behavioral outcomes.

Home-based interventions addressing ADLs and IADLs not only affect outcomes for the client but also may have an effect on the caregiver. Dooley and Hinojosa (2004), in a Level II pretest–posttest control group design, found that an in-home occupational therapy assessment followed by a review of recommendations with an occupational therapist improved the quality of life and reduced caregiver burden for 40 caregivers of memory disorder clinic participants. A Level I randomized control study of a home-based intervention known as TAP (Tailored Activity Program), designed to promote leisure time activity, found positive effects on the caregiver in managing problem behaviors and promoting independent activity engagement for the client (Gitlin et al., 2008).

In the area of ADLs, studies have been performed on the effects of graded assistance and positive reinforcement on mealtime behaviors and food textures. A mealtime program that used family-style versus prepared plates was found to increase dining participation in a Level IV single-subject design study (Altus et al., 2002). Their findings support the use of praise by dining assistants to prevent excess disability and increase participation when the client is capable. Beattie, Algase, and Song (2004) found, in a Level III before–after study with three participants, that increased communication strategies and positive social reinforcement reduced mealtime wandering and increased food intake. Van Ort and Phillips (1995), in a Level III one-group, repeated-measures design, compared a behavioral approach (cues and reinforcement) to a contextual approach (self-feeding setup and positive atmosphere) and found that both approaches promoted self-feeding. Food textures were studied in this Level III before–after study, with softer food texture resulting in increased food intake (Boylston, Ryan, Brown, & Westfall, 1995). These studies, albeit limited by small sample sizes and weak statistical measures, support the use of behavioral strategies to promote self-feeding in the later stages of the disease in residential care.

Some studies have explored the use of physical and cognitive assistive devices in promoting participation with people with cognitive impairment. Nochajski, Tomita, and Mann (1996), in a Level III pretest–posttest study, found that people with higher cognitive status were more likely to use and express satisfaction with assistive devices (MMSE 15 to 23) than were people with lower cognitive status. The challenges to new learning and progressive decline in thinking may influence proper or continued use of physical and cognitive aides. In a follow-up Level III study, the use of physical devices was found to decline as the disease progressed (Yang, Mann, Nochajski, & Tomita, 1997). More research needs to be conducted on the use and effectiveness of assistive devices and dementia.

Leisure or recreational interventions were found to promote social participation during family visits using sensorimotor activities. Buettner (1999), in a Level III study, used 30 recreational items for nursing home residents in a dementia unit. After family caregiver education, the family members incorporated these activities during family visits and found 23 of the activities to be therapeutically valuable. In a follow-up study, the recreational items were found to increase the number of visits and satisfaction with visits and to reduce the agitation of the resident (Colling & Buettner, 2002). This study promotes the use of objects, adapted and designed to the client's cognitive level, to facilitate participation in activities. Mentioned previously as a home-based intervention, the TAP program is designed to tailor activities to the client's capacity to increase involvement in activities. It was successful in engaging the person in activity with reported high client and caregiver satisfaction (Gitlin et al., 2008). Crispi and Heitner (2002), in a Level IV descriptive study, developed 10 kits based on ability levels for family members to use during visits. They found that 6 kits were useful and that puzzles and reminiscence kits contributed to a higher quality of visits than card games or a "sounds of the past" activity. Politis and colleagues (2004), in a Level I randomized controlled group study, compared a kit-based activity intervention with a one-to-one conversation intervention. They found no difference

between the two groups in the effects on apathy and behavior but did find within-group improvements on quality-of-life measures for the control group. Chung (2004), in a Level III cross-sectional study, explored activity patterns of people in the mild, moderate, and severe stage of dementia. She found significant differences in the amount of time in therapeutic/leisure, ADLs, and mobility and interaction among the groups. She also found that well-being was correlated to activities that had the potential for interaction.

Research findings from other disciplines can provide information related to leisure participation. In a Level III study, Clair and Ebberts (1997) explored the effects of music therapy on the relationship between caregivers and care receivers and found that music improved visits and participation when playing rhythm instruments compared with conversing. In an art therapy study, clients increased their sustained attention time during a watercolor and acrylic painting activity (Rentz, 2002). Specific measures were not included in this Level IV descriptive study. More rigorous and targeted research is needed on leisure programming; occupational therapy practitioners may be involved with the development of music and art activities in an adult day services program for people with dementia.

Intervention Performance Skills and Performance Patterns

Performance skills, defined as motor, sensory–perceptual, cognitive, emotional, and social skills, are affected in people with Alzheimer's disease. The degree of impact follows the stage approach, with skills declining gradually and somewhat predictably over the course of the disease. Declining motor and praxis skills contribute to an increased risk of falls and the eventual need for mobility devices. Disturbing changes in perceptual skills result in getting lost in a familiar environment and the eventual nonrecognition of family members. Emotional regulation weakens as people become increasingly difficult to understand, precipitating behavioral agitation and, ultimately, catastrophic reactions. The ability to communicate declines, and caregivers must find alternative methods to uncover the needs the client is attempting to resolve. Intervention with performance skills may involve prevention (e.g., a fall prevention program, validation therapy) or compensation (e.g., enrolling in a Safe Return or Comfort Zone program [Alzheimer's Association, 2008, 2009b] or feeding program). Behavioral management programs can provide the caregiver with strategies to divert negative emotional reactions and to guide the client in a positive direction.

Clients with short-term memory deficits draw from premorbid abilities and skills embedded in long-term or procedural memory. These *splinter skills* are remarkable and unique to each person, often related to past routines and habits. The objective of the occupational profile is to identify a person's unique skills and abilities, along with the areas of limitation. The strengths are then incorporated into the plan of intervention to guide recommendations for meaningful, individualized activities.

Performance patterns refer to the habits, routines, roles, and rituals that structure the daily life of an individual. With Alzheimer's disease, habits may disintegrate (both good and bad habits), routines and rituals are affected, and roles are redefined. Disruption in routines can lead to catastrophic reactions and caregiver stress. Interventions include habit training along with positive reinforcement and consistent reassurance. Interventions targeting performance patterns have focused on structuring daytime activity and routines of sleep and toileting.

Evidence for Intervention With Performance Skills and Performance Patterns

Interventions that target performance skills are designed to change abilities to improve occupational performance. Programs that target motor and praxis skills have been studied to determine the effects on cognitive function, behavior, and physiological indexes. Heyn (2003), in a Level III pretest–posttest

study, found that a structured group multisensory exercise session 3 times a week for 8 weeks increased engagement in activity, improved mood for some participants, and increased resting heart rate. Further research on the use of exercise to affect performance skills is needed.

There has been a surge of research into falls prevention programs for the elderly population and a few limited number of studies specific to people with dementia. These studies examined falls prevention programs aimed at caregiver and staff education, physical training for balance and strength, or a multifaceted approach including components of education and physical training. Educational falls prevention programs have demonstrated success in Level III pretest–posttest studies in reducing the number of falls by high-risk people with dementia (Detweiler, Kim, & Taylor, 2005; Mackintosh & Sheppard, 2005; Savage & Matheis-Kraft, 2001).

One Level I randomized controlled trial study that relied on a falls risk manual for staff training along with a falls risk assessment did not reduce falls in a residential care facility, with 50% of the population reported as having dementia (Kerse, Butler, Robinson, & Todd, 2004). This finding indicates a staff training method for falls prevention may not have an effect on falls-related outcomes. Savage and Matheis-Kraft (2001), in a Level II pretest–posttest study, found that an intense, falls-focused training program for certified nursing assistants decreased the number, but not the severity, of falls in eight residents with dementia. Multifactorial falls prevention interventions to reduce incidence of falls have been less conclusive (Jensen et al., 2003; 2004; Oliver et al., 2007; Shaw et al., 2003). All studies were Level I randomized controlled trials, except for Oliver and colleagues (2007), which was a systematic review. What studies did find was that the multifactorial approach, which may include staff education, environmental adjustment, exercise, drug review, aids, hip protectors, and postfall problem-solving conferences, work better for people with higher levels of cognition (Jensen et al., 2003) and in hospital versus home care settings (Oliver et al., 2007). A Level I systematic review indicated that the results of physical strengthening programs for people with dementia are also inconclusive (Hauer, Becker, Lindemann, & Beyer, 2006). Although studies showed favorable outcomes, including improvement in balance, walking speed, flexibility, and strength, they did not demonstrate an effect on the fall rate. This area deserves further study.

Stenvall and colleagues (2007), in a Level I randomized controlled trial, studied an orthopedic, postoperative, multidisciplinary intervention program for people with and without dementia. The program included occupational and physical therapy both in hospital and home visits. They found in the dementia group there were fewer fallers and fewer total falls. This finding supports active involvement in occupational therapy for fall prevention after femoral neck fracture.

Programs have been implemented to increase security for people with dementia who have altered perceptual skills. Wandering, way-finding, or exit-seeking behavior can be one of the most stress-provoking symptoms for family or facility caregivers to monitor (Dickinson, McLain-Kark, & Marshall-Baker, 1995). Visual interventions in the form of murals, posters, and concealment of doors or door knobs have been used to divert way-finding (exiting) behaviors (Kincaid & Peacock, 2003; Level III). A cloth barrier over the door and concealment of a door knob was found to reduce exiting attempts for residents on a dementia care unit in two Level III studies (Dickinson et al., 1995; Namazi, Rosner, & Calkins, 1989). To measure the effects of barrier heights in an activities room, Namazi and Johnson (1992a; Level III) measured distractibility in high versus low barriers. High barriers reduced distractions, indicating the need to reduce auditory stimuli in large common areas of a facility used for activity programming for people with dementia. In a Level IV single-subject design study, Cohen-Mansfield and Werner (1998) installed a nature scene and a home-and-people scene in a corridor of the nursing home to reduce pacing and wandering. They found no statistical significance on most measures, although the study did report an impact on pacing behavior, time residents sat to view the scenes, and

resident's level of agitation. A way-finding program was tested with nursing home residents with dementia to enable them to find their way to the dining room in a Level I randomized controlled trial (McGilton, Rivera, & Dawson, 2003). The program of backward chaining, communication, and use of location maps demonstrated results only for a short time. The program appeared to decrease agitation initially, but the agitated behavior reappeared after 3 months.

Structural environments have been studied to determine whether an L-shaped, an H-shaped, or a corridor design would have a different impact on behavioral reactions in residents with dementia in a Level II nonrandomized controlled study (Elmståhl, Annerstedt, & Åhlund, 1997). The results indicated that those in the corridor design had more time disorientation than those in the L-shaped design over a 6-month period. In addition, those in the corridor had significant reductions in identity during a 12-month period as opposed to no similar changes in the L-shaped or H-shaped groups. Another study examined locked and unlocked exit doors. It found that people with dementia increase unwanted behaviors when encountering a locked door, although significance was not determined in this Level III study (Namazi & Johnson, 1992b). Structural environments have the potential as an area for future research in determining the impact of environmental design on behavioral and occupational performance.

In examining signage to stimulate way-finding abilities in residential facilities, Passini, Pigot, Rainville, and Tetreault (2000) explored staff perceptions of the effectiveness of visual cues in a Level IV multiple case study. Results were inconclusive, although staff reported that the use of pictographs warranted further research. Gibson and colleagues (2004), in a Level IV descriptive study, used a new resident orientation protocol to orient residents to their own rooms and reduce intrusion in others' rooms. They reported that 100% of residents found their own room with three repetitions of the orientation and used multiple environmental cues; those intruding in other residents' rooms appeared to be seeking social interaction. A Level II nonrandomized controlled trial compared a special care unit in which residents had unrestricted mobility to a regular controlled mobility unit. The results indicated that that greater freedom of movement led to less disruptive and more social behaviors as demonstrated by fewer catastrophic reactions in the special care unit (Swanson, Maas, & Buckwalter, 1994). Measures of cognition and functional abilities showed no difference between the two groups.

Difficulties with emotional regulation lead to behavior management problems both at home and within a residential facility during the middle and later stages of the disease. Various types of sensory stimulation have been studied to reduce agitation and manage difficult behaviors and to improve overall well-being. Auditory interventions highlight the use of music to stimulate well-being and counteract time spent in meaningless activity (Sherratt, Thornton, & Hatton, 2004). Gotell, Brown, and Ekman (2003), in a phenomenological study, found that background music and caregiver singing appeared to promote competence in morning grooming activities, improve sensory awareness, and enhance caregiver interactions. In a Level II study comparing live music to recorded music and no music, both the live and recorded music were effective in increasing well-being (Sherratt et al., 2004).

Koss and Gilmore (1998) studied ambient light to reduce agitation during the later afternoon hours, sometimes referred to as *sundowner's syndrome.* In a Level III before–after study, they found that increasing light intensity reduced agitation significantly and increased food consumption at mealtimes (Koss & Glimore, 1998). Enhancing light intensity was a relatively easy modification to implement for the outcomes identified. A Level IV case series of an optical intervention with people dually diagnosed with ocular pathology and dementia was conducted by Pankow, Pliskin, and Luchins (1996). They found reduced hallucinations reported by all three participants when visual aids were used (telescopic devises for distance, high powered lenses for near vision, and prisms for peripheral vision).

Sensory integration intervention has been used to reduce agitation and difficult behaviors in people with dementia. A Level I randomized controlled study of standardized sensory integration sessions (3 45-min sessions over 10 weeks) with people with dementia found a decrease in disruptive behaviors and caregiver reactions, as well as an improvement in function. When adjusting for covariates, however, using an analysis of covariance, no significant effect on behaviors was found (Robichaud, Hebert, & Desrosiers, 1994).

Snoezelen is a multisensory approach using a specially designed room to manipulate the mood and behavior of people with dementia. There are increased costs and staff time associated with the intervention. Chung and Lai (2002) conducted a Level I systematic review and concluded that there was limited evidence to support or refute this approach and that performance outcomes have not been established. A Level IV single case design study compared Snoezelen to music relaxation sessions and found improved mood, affect, and behavior in a positive way with Snoezelen, resulting in a higher incidence of happiness (Pinkney, 1997). In other studies, Snoezelen has been found to reduce agitation immediately after the session but without sustainability (van Diepen et al., 2002; Level I randomized controlled trial), reduce agitation equally as effective as a reminiscence group (Baillon et al., 2004, 2005; Level I randomized controlled trials), and affect deviant behaviors better than an activity group (Baker, Dowling, Wareing, Dawson, & Assey, 1997; Level I randomized controlled trial), but these studies have not linked the intervention to occupational performance.

Lantz, Buchalter, and McBee (1997), in a Level II study, found that agitation was reduced in both the intervention and control groups by increasing client self-awareness using meditation, guided imagery, relaxation, and body awareness, although greater reductions were reported in the intervention group. Rosswurm (1990), in a Level I study, used attention-focusing groups and relaxation with people with dementia for improving performance on visual exercises. These performance skill interventions that focused on improving a particular skill, however, did not carry over to occupational performance. Although the study designs lacked rigor, mindfulness-based interventions warrant further research with this population.

Cognitive interventions for improving cognitive skills have had limited success because of the declining abilities of the person with Alzheimer's disease. Spector and colleagues (2003), in a Level I randomized controlled trial, added cognitive stimulation therapy (information processing) to the task adaptation and found it improved cognition and quality of life but did not improve functional ability in communication or affect levels of anxiety or depression. Interventions to improve communication and social skills have not been studied extensively. Further outcomes research is needed to investigate interventions targeting performance skills with people with dementia and, specifically, Alzheimer's type. The gap in research is, in measuring the effects of the interventions on occupational performance as it is affected by behavior, cognition, and perception.

There is weak but positive evidence that supports the structuring of routines to compensate for memory loss in the early stages of the disease and to remove structure in routines in managing challenging behaviors in the later stages of the disease. Nygård and Johansson (2001) used time aid interventions (adaptive clocks, special calendars) to assist people with memory loss in managing daily routines and schedules. Using a qualitative method, they found that two of the five participants were able to address their problems related to planning appointments. In a qualitative study, Skovdahl, Kihlgren, and Kihlgren (2003) found that routines constrained staff response to clients during a showering activity. The need to complete the task appeared to take priority over the person's negative reactions to the task. Likewise, Donovan and Dupuis (2000), in a qualitative study, found that residents preferred to follow their own pattern of routines for daily care, and flexibility in routine was perceived as a positive element in the dementia care unit.

Studies have been conducted to measure the effectiveness of establishing routines for voiding. The use of *timed voiding* (regularly scheduled), *habit retraining* (setting up a voiding schedule on the basis of observation), and *prompted voiding* (asking and assisting frequently) have been examined and incorporated as standard practice in managing incontinence with dementia as reported in a Level I evidence-based review (Doody et al., 2001). The evidence is inconclusive for habit retraining and timed voiding in Level I systematic reviews (Ostaszkiewicz, Johnston, & Roe, 2004a, 2004b) but supportive of prompted voiding (Eustice, Roe, & Paterson, 2000; Level I systematic review; Skelly & Flint, 1995; Level V narrative review).

Interventions to establish sleep routines have been found to be useful in long-term facilities. These multimodal interventions included participating in daily walking and physical activity, eliminating daytime sleeping, taking part in light therapy, and establishing nighttime routines. In a Level I randomized controlled trial, Alessi and colleagues (2005) reported a significant decrease in mean awakening length (minutes) and a significant decrease (46%) in observed daytime sleeping in the intervention group, along with significant increases in participation in social and physical activities. There was no significant change in nighttime total sleep, percentage of sleep, or number of awakenings and no difference noted with levels of agitation or assistance in eating or drinking. In Level I randomized controlled trials for a home care multimodal program, McCurry and colleagues (2003) achieved consistency of bedtime (83% intervention group vs. 38% control group), consistency of rising time (96% vs. 59%), reduction of napping (70% vs. 28%), and participation in a walking program (86% vs. 7%). All of these differences were statistically significant. In a 2005 study by the same team of researchers, caregivers reported significant differences in the intervention group in nighttime awake time, with fewer awakenings of less duration and more daily exercise and lower depression ratings (measured by Revised Memory and Behavioral Problems Checklist).

Intervention Contexts and Environments

Contextual or environmental interventions include environmental modifications, caregiver education and training programs, and access to community resources. Many of the contextual interventions overlap because caregivers make the modifications as part of a larger, multistrategic intervention plan. For instance, in a case of wandering or way finding, an environmental modification may be to install outside movement sensors and training the caregiver in approaches to guide the client away from and to secure restricted areas. The standard for occupational therapy intervention is to consider the context and environment along with the person and the task and the interaction among these dimensions.

Caregiver education and training is an integral part of occupational therapy intervention for people with Alzheimer's disease. Family interventions include home-based, outpatient, or institutional-based care protocols that can be applied during family visits. Caregiver education includes training staff and paid caregivers in managing daily cares for the client. Studies examining the effectiveness of caregiver education programs are finding success in alleviating caregiver stress and improving client care. In a meta-analysis of caregiver interventions, Sörensen, Pinquart, and Duberstein (2002) found decreased caregiver burden, depression, and care receiver symptoms and improved subjective well-being, caregiver satisfaction, and increased ability and knowledge, although dementia caregivers had smaller effects than other groups. Teri, McCurry, Logsdon, and Gibbons (2005) investigated the effectiveness of community consultants in educating family caregivers in behavioral approaches to mood and problem behaviors. They found that education provided by trained consultants reduced frequency and severity of problem behaviors and improved quality of life for the client. This finding indicates that occupational therapy could also be effective in using a consultant approach in guiding family caregivers in treatment protocols.

Evidence for Intervention With Contexts and Environments

Strong evidence supports the implementation of environmental strategies in interventions for people with dementia. In a pivotal occupational therapy study, Graff and colleagues (2006), in a Level I randomized controlled trial, found that 10 sessions of community occupational therapy intervention, based on compensatory and environmental modifications, improved daily functioning in ADL and IADL performance and reduced the burden of care for the primary caregiver. The research group further found that occupational therapy intervention was a cost-effective approach in treating community-dwelling people with cognitive involvement on the basis of the same data (Graff et al., 2008). This widely reported, rigorous study supports increased attention to the role of occupational therapy in the community with this population. Other studies have less rigor but can inform practice, providing a variety of strategies for managing behaviors related to declining cognition in both community and facility settings.

Nolan and colleagues (2001) conducted a Level IV single-subject design/multiple baseline to determine whether door signage and a photo increased room-finding abilities. Room finding improved for the three study participants. Although the sample size was small, personal cues are an inexpensive method to increase ability to independently navigate the environment.

Environmental interventions include activity programs and alteration of the space where the programs occur. Opie, Rosewarne, and O'Connor (1999) conducted a Level I systematic review of nonpharmacological strategies to alleviate behavioral disturbances. The results of the review indicated there is evidence to support the efficacy of activity programs, music, behavior therapy, light therapy, caregiver education, and changes to the physical environment. The evidence was inconclusive for the support of multidisciplinary teams, massage, and aromatherapy. Although most studies lacked rigor because of small sample sizes, the evidence does support continued research on these types of interventions. Whall and colleagues (1997), in a Level II nonrandomized controlled trial, studied the effect of natural environments on agitated and aggressive behavior during a bathing/showering task. They found that adverse behaviors decreased with bird songs, babbling brooks, bright pictures, and favorite foods.

Other studies measured the outcomes of activity programming using a small group, individualized approach (Montessori-based) versus a large group (Orsulic-Jeras, Judge, & Camp, 2000; Level II within-subject nonrandomized controlled trial) and the type of activities, common use materials (Montessori) versus passive (TV, coloring, and drawing; Vance & Johns, 2002; Level II within-subject nonrandomized controlled trial). These studies, although single-facility studies, do point to the prospect that factors in designing programs can affect attention, memory, object permanence, pleasure, and, indirectly, occupational performance. Orsulic-Jeras and colleagues (2000) found significantly more constructive engagement in the intervention group using individually tailored activities with familiar materials from the everyday environment of the residents.

Interventions affecting the social context include those actions that impact the client's social network, targeting the caregiver directly as the recipient of service and the client indirectly. These interventions are generally in the form of caregiver education and training. Four occupational therapy interventions have been studied that demonstrate how caregiver intervention can positively influence factors in the care of people with dementia. Gitlin and colleagues (2005), in the Level I randomized controlled trial REACH 2 (Resources for Enhancing Alzheimer's Caregivers Health) program, found that six occupational therapy sessions (5 90-min home visits and 1 telephone session) improved caregiver skills, decreased client need for assistance, and reduced behavioral occurrences. The intervention effects were noted in a 6-month follow-up. Gitlin and colleagues (2008) studied the effects of the TAP, which focused on selecting and customizing activities to match capabilities and train-

ing caregivers in the use of activities (6 90-min home visits and 2 15-min phone contacts). Caregivers reported reduced frequency of problem behaviors and greater activity engagement, and the effects endured at a 4-month follow-up. The primary focus of the Graff and colleagues (2006) study was caregiver training in environmental modifications and compensatory strategies to improve ADL performance. The results of the study indicates that clients functioned significantly better in daily living skills, and caregivers reported greater confidence. At a 12-week follow-up, the effects of the interventions were still significant. Dooley and Hinojosa (2004), in a Level I randomized controlled trial, found that training caregivers to cue, break down tasks, give step-by-step instructions, structure routines, and promote activities was effective in increasing quality of life and promoting independence in self-care. These studies specifically focused on occupational performance outcome measures that provide strong evidence of the benefits resulting from caregiver education and training.

Most studies that focus primarily on the caregiver come from disciplines outside of occupational therapy, but they can inform practice that incorporates caregiver training methods. Many studies have focused on interventions to alleviate caregiver reactions to caregiving, measuring outcomes such as burden, stress, satisfaction, and depression. A Level I meta-analysis of these interventions (support groups, education, psychoeducation, counseling, respite care) showed that few had significant effects on caregiver burden (2 of 27 interventions; Acton & Kang, 2001). Another Level I meta-analysis of interventions (caregiver and family counseling, education, client involvement, support groups, stress management programs) showed a modest but significant benefit for knowledge, psychological morbidity, coping skills, and social support (Brodaty, Green, & Koschera, 2003).

Other studies showed that the effect on reducing caregiver burden through caregiver interventions remains mixed, ranging from no impact (Brodaty et al., 2003; Peacock & Forbes, 2003; systematic review) to reductions in stress, depression, and burden (Hepburn,

Tornatore, Center, & Ostwald, 2001; Level I randomized controlled trial; Mittelman, Roth, Clay, & Haley, 2007; Level I randomized controlled trial). A systematic review of the literature by Cooke, McNally, Mulligan, Harrison, and Newman (2001) found little evidence to warrant education and counseling for improving caregiver well-being. In fact, one Level I randomized controlled study reported that educational materials for client behavior management given to caregivers resulted in worse outcomes and increased risk for depression (Burns, Nichols, Martindale-Adams, Graney, & Lummus, 2003). By contrast, outcomes of an occupational therapy intervention focusing on client outcomes (Graff et al., 2007) showed that caregiver quality of life, mood, and health status demonstrated improvements.

Respite care that allows the caregiver reprieve from caregiving responsibilities did not demonstrate benefits or adverse effects on the caregiver in a Level I systematic review (Lee & Cameron, 2004). By contrast, adult day service programs were found to support caregivers in alleviating care-related stress and enhancing caregiver opportunity for social and recreational activities (Schacke & Zank, 2006; Level II nonrandomized controlled trial).

Another outcome of interest in light of the high costs of institutional care is delayed institutional placements or nursing home admissions. Studies that examined the effects of caregiver intervention on institutional placement reported some favorable effects. Mittelman, Haley, Clay, and Roth (2006) found caregiver counseling, caregiver support groups, and telephone access for support delayed nursing home placement and improved caregiver satisfaction in a Level I randomized controlled trial. They found multiple factors that predicted nursing home placement, including increased severity of dementia, poorer caregiver physical health, lower satisfaction with social support, greater frequency of memory and behavior problems, more symptoms of depression, and higher caregiver burden. In an earlier study, Mittelman and colleagues (1996) found that multidimensional caregiver support could delay nursing home placement by 329 days. A Level I systematic review of the literature

that included 25 studies (Smits et al., 2007) revealed that combined programs for caregivers result in positive outcomes, including delaying long-term care. Alternatives to institutional placement and the effects on caregiver and client well-being deserve continued study.

The use of technology, including telephone network interventions and weekly phone conversations, has been studied to determine the effects on health outcomes for caregivers. In a Level I systematic literature review, Thompson and colleagues (2007) reported that group-based supportive interventions positively affected caregiver psychological morbidity, whereas technology and individual-based interventions did not demonstrate effectiveness. By contrast, Bank, Argüelles, Rubert, Eisdorfer, and Czaja (2006), in a Level III pretest–posttest design study, found that telephone support groups (18 months) with in-home family therapy (12 months) increased caregiver report of knowledge and skills as caregivers (73%), knowledge about memory disorders (70%), community resources (68%), improved relationships with family members (62%), and increased willingness to participate in a community-based support group (51%).

Interventions affecting the temporal context are limited in number. Kovach and colleagues (2004), in a Level I randomized controlled trial, studied the effectiveness of the BACE (Balancing, Arousal, Controls, Excesses) intervention in decreasing agitation in people with dementia. BACE is a daily activity schedule that balances the time a person is in a high-arousal and low-arousal state. Kovach and colleagues (2004) found that balancing arousal states contributed to decreased agitation. This finding indicates that a person's temporal context or daily schedule may be altered or adjusted to affect behavioral reactions.

Intervention Activity Demands

Occupational therapy intervention includes modifying activity demands to meet client capabilities, interests, and personality style. Few studies measure the effectiveness of intervention on modifying activity demands. According to the AOTA (2002), *activity demands* are "the aspects of an activity which include the objects, space, social demands, sequencing or timing, required actions, and required underlying body functions and body structure needed to carry out the activity" (p. 624). This intervention includes altering the materials, approach to the task, method of completing the task, assistance provided, or expectations of the product or result. The goal of intervention is to increase the supports (external contextual factors) to mimic the rate of cognitive decline (internal client factors) for optimal successful participation (see Figure 4).

Verbal and nonverbal cues by a caregiver are considered an external support and one of the ways of altering activity demands. As the disease progresses, the amount of monitoring increases from periodic monitoring to occasional monitoring to frequent monitoring. Likewise, supervision increases over time. The task may initially require a single demonstration, progressing to multiple demonstrations. Cueing is modified from general instructions to specific instructions, abstract to concrete, multistep to single step. The caregiver initially assists with portions of a task to later assisting with the full task. In later stages of the disease, when the client is unable to physically participate, the client may observe the activity, gradually reducing observation time to accommodate attention span.

Task adaptations are another method of altering activity demands. The task can be adapted by reducing the number of task objects or simplifying the procedures, setting up the task, completing portions of the task before active client involvement, or controlling the environment. If the client can no longer participate in the task, client observation is a form of passive involvement.

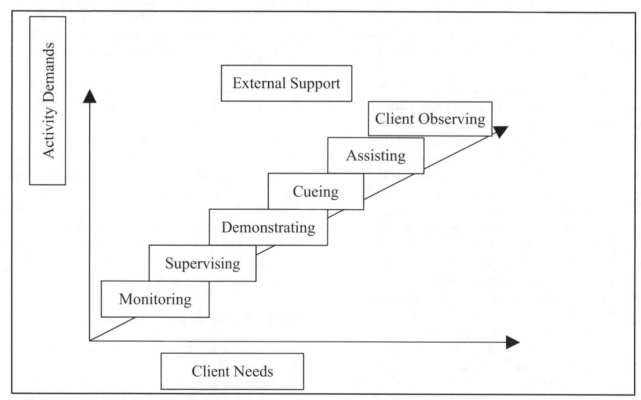

Figure 4. Progression of external supports to meet client needs for assistance.

Evidence on Intervention for Activity Demands

Occupational therapy intervention, specifically, modifying activity demands, has been shown to be effective in maintaining independence over time for people with Alzheimer's disease. Adjusting activity demands for mealtime with behavioral prompts and positive reinforcement (Coyne & Hoskins, 1997; Level I randomized controlled trial) and environmental prompts such as music, dining setting, and altering personnel (Watson & Green, 2006; Level I systematic review) contributed to greater mealtime independence. Rogers and colleagues (1999), in a Level III study, found that habit training and skill elicitation (graded assistance to elicit the highest level of performance) increased independence in performing dressing tasks, improved participation in assisted dressing, decreased disruptive behaviors, and increased appropriate requests for help with nursing home residents with dementia. Kolanowski (2001), in a Level I randomized crossover design, found that tailoring activities to the client's skill level and personal interests increased time spent on task and displays of positive affect, although it did not affect participation.

Effects of modification of activity demands were shown to persist over time. In a follow-up of an intensive 2-day feeding program, effects were present after 7 days (Coyne & Hoskins, 1997). Likewise, Graff and colleagues (2006) measured a 5-week occupational therapy intervention after 3 months and found increased effects on daily functioning still present. In an individually designed activity program (TAP), administered through 6 90-minute home visits and 2 15-minute telephone contacts, caregivers reported greater activity involvement and reduced problem behaviors than the control group after 4 months (Gitlin et al., 2008; Level I randomized controlled trial). Although these studies support interventions that modify activity demands for people with dementing diseases, more studies specific to clients with Alzheimer's disease are needed.

Intervention Client Factors

Interventions related to client factors include those that motivate an individual to engage in occupational performance because they match a person's values, beliefs, and spirituality or personal quest for meaning. Interventions targeted toward client factors also include those that affect the physiological (i.e., cardiovascular, respiratory, endocrine) and anatomical structures (skeletal and circulatory). These interventions are designed to enhance the sensory (visual, auditory, tactile, vestibular) and motor systems (strength, balance, coordination) and cognition. Numerous attempts have been made to use interventions directed toward client factors to influence difficult behaviors, increase functional independence, and reduce caregiver burden. Although the intent is to alter client factors directly, many are environmental approaches designed to regulate or stimulate sensory input or compensate for declining abilities. Many of these interventions were previously discussed under environmental modifications with the evidence presented.

Multisensory interventions include programs like Snoezelen, which control sensory input for the individual to alter mood or behavior. Music or auditory regulation of the environment includes reducing extraneous noise like television, intercom systems, buzzers, and alarms. Visual environments such as colors, lighting, space designs, elimination of mirrors, or personnel cues have been used institutionally and incorporated into architectural planning of new environments for dementia care units. Programs like the Eden alternative, a nature-themed environment with plants, animals, and children, have been created with favorable results reported by those living in the facility. Tactile interventions include Healing Touch, a trained intervention to reduce agitation or distress. Rocking chairs or gliders that provide vestibular input are used to subdue clients during nighttime insomnias.

Cognitive interventions include reality orientation and reminiscence. These popular programs stimulate thinking and memory and bring temporary enjoyment from the engagement in group activity but have a limited long-term effect on cognitive abilities. Cognitive approaches early in the disease involve the use of memory aides, schedules, calendars, systems for compensating for memory loss, and habit training. Although the adage "use it or lose it" makes sense with aging people, cognitive exercises do little to counteract progressive cognitive decline in Alzheimer's disease. Even so, cognitive stimulation can be beneficial in that it reminds family members that the client should remain involved in daily conversation and thinking as long as frustration is minimized.

Mobility skill training has been used to improve ambulation and reduce falls. Interventions that target motor skills include aerobic and strength training exercise programs that are indirectly related to cognitive abilities but directly related to client well-being. As previously mentioned in the falls section, the goal of targeted physical activity is to maintain safe gait and balance skills further into the course of the disease when falls risk increases. Mobility skill training also promotes continued activity engagement and counteracts occupational deprivation.

Although many studies have focused on altering client factors through environmental modifications, most have minimal or limited effect as an intervention approach. The nature of the disease is that body functions and structures are gradually altering, creating barriers to occupational performance. To promote quality of life, interventions should incorporate the person's innate desire to achieve through selection of activities that motivate and challenge the person, accommodating the changing ability levels.

Summary of the Evidence-Based Literature Review

The evidence-based reviews included 129 articles. Of these articles, 69 were at the highest level of evidence as Level I studies. In addition, 12 were Level II studies, 29 were Level III studies, 13 were Level IV studies, and 1 was a Level V study. Six qualitative studies also were incorporated into the review. All studies included in the review, as well as those not specifically described in the evidence-based literature review section of this Practice Guideline, are summarized, critically appraised, and cited in full in the evidence tables in Appendix E. The evidence tables also include implications for occupational therapy practice. Readers are encouraged to read the full articles for more details. Further recommendations for occupational therapy practice for people with Alzheimer's disease can be found in Table 10. The recommendations are based on the strength of the evidence for a given topic in combination with the expert opinion of the review authors and content experts reviewing this Guideline. The strength of the evidence is determined by the number of articles included in a given topic, the study design, and limitations of those articles. Recommendation criteria are based on standard language developed by the U.S. Preventive Services Task Force of the Agency for Health Care Research and Quality. More information regarding these criteria can be found at http://www.ahrq.gov/clinic/uspstf/standard.htm.

The evidence-based literature review focused on the effectiveness of interventions in areas of occupation (ADLs, IADLs, leisure, social), environmental and contextual modifications, establishment of performance patterns including routines, performance skills focusing on perception, alteration of activity demands, and fall prevention. The recommendations for intervention planning in ADLs point out the need to tailor the intervention to the stage of the disease, specifically, using assistive devices in the early stages of the disease (Nochajski et al., 1996), focusing on modifying or adapting ADLs in the middle stages of the disease (Altus et al., 2002), and providing caregiver training and behavioral interventions in the later stages of the disease (Beattie et al., 2004). Studies examining IADLs focused on the setting for service delivery with success in compensatory and environmental strategies in community and home-based interventions in the early stages of the disease (Dooley & Hinojosa, 2004; Graff et al., 2007) and programmatic interventions in dementia care units in the later stages of the disease (Fitzsimmons &

Table 10. Recommendations for Occupational Therapy Interventions for Clients With Alzheimer's Disease

	Recommended	No Recommendation	Not Recommended
Areas of Occupation	Client-centered occupational therapy identifying occupational performance issues and helping clients implement compensatory and environmental strategies for people with mild to moderate dementia (A)	Reminiscence activities (I)	
	Client-centered activities (e.g., leisure) tailored to the person with dementia (B)		
	Multifaceted interventions (including removal of physical restraints, fall alarm, exercise, change in environment) to prevent falls (A for hospital and geriatric hospital settings, C for community and nursing home settings)		
	Physical training (gait, strengthening, balance, and flexibility) to prevent falls for older adults with cognitive impairments (B)		
	Regular therapeutic cooking group for residents (B)		
	Direct training that includes errorless learning, memory training, and ADL training (C)		
	At the early stages of the disease, assessment and training on the use of cognitive and physical assistive technology (C)		
	At later stages of the disease, adjusting food texture, and providing occupation-based and client-centered strategies to maintain weight and reduce wandering (C)		
Performance Skills			
Perception	Attention-focusing group to improve visual matching and activities (B)	Snoezelen (I)	
	Music, body awareness, and mobility/functional training (B)	Sensory integration (I)	
	Use of live or recorded music (C)		
	Use of multisensory environments (C)		
Fall Prevention	Multifaceted interventions (including removal of physical restraints, fall alarm, exercise, change in environment) to prevent falls (A for hospital and geriatric hospital settings, C for community and nursing home settings)		
	Physical training (gait, strengthening, balance, and flexibility) to prevent falls for older adults with cognitive impairments (B)		
Routines	Sleep routines and sleep hygiene strategies to improve daytime activities and nighttime sleeping (A)		
	Prompted voiding strategies for toileting (B)		
	Timed voiding and habit retraining strategies for toileting (C)		
	General use of client-centered routines (C)		
	Skill elicitation and individualized behavioral interventions for habit training during ADL performance (C)		

(continued)

Table 10. Recommendations for Occupational Therapy Interventions for Clients With Alzheimer's Disease (cont.)

	Recommended	No Recommendation	Not Recommended
Context and Environment			
Physical Environment	Intervention provided by occupational therapy practitioner that emphasizes the use of compensatory and environmental strategies that include cueing and step-by-step instructions (A) Multifaceted interventions (including removal of physical restraints, fall alarm, exercise, change in environment) to prevent falls (A for hospital and geriatric hospital settings, C for community and nursing home settings) Changes to the physical environment such as activity therapy, music, and natural environment simulations (B) Use of Montessori materials that incorporate aesthetically pleasing materials from the environment (B) Use of an schedule to balance high-arousal and low-arousal states (B) Increased lighting at mealtime (C) Changes to doors and exits (doors unlocked, concealment of knobs, portable visual barriers, and murals to disguise doorknobs) (C) At the early stages of the disease, assessment and training on the use of cognitive and physical assistive technology (C)	Snoezelen (I) Massage and aromatherapy (I) Bright light therapy (I) Enhancement of corridors and other changes in environmental design in residential facilities (I) Units that emphasize the control of sensory stimulation, use of soothing music, and a decrease in traffic (I) Signs and photographs outside residents' rooms to assist with way finding (I)	
Person–Caregiver	Occupational therapy sessions that provide caregivers with education, problem solving, technical skills (task simplification, communication), and simple home modifications (A) Caregiver interventions combining counseling and support groups (A) Caregiver interventions that combine education, case management, client involvement, stress management, and training (A) Interventions taking place in the client's home (B) Customized activity-based interventions in conjunction with instructions to caregivers (B) Participation in a support group (B) Technology-mediated support groups (B) Day care for people with Alzheimer's disease (C)	Respite care (I)	Interventions focusing only on the behavior of the person with dementia (D) Interventions focusing only on knowledge of dementia (D)
Activity Demands	Intervention provided by occupational therapy practitioner that emphasizes the use of compensatory and environmental strategies that include cueing and step-by-step instructions (A) Interventions during feeding that include consistent verbal prompts from carer, reinforcement for eating, use of music during dining, and changes in meal presentation (A) Skill elicitation and individualized behavioral interventions for habit training during ADL performance (C) Activity selection on the basis of personal style of client (C) Cognitive stimulation therapy with adapted daily tasks matched to ability level (C)		

Note. Recommendation criteria are based on standard language Agency for Healthcare Research and Quality (2009). Suggested recommendations are based on the available evidence and content experts' opinions. ADL = activities of daily living.

A—Strongly recommend that occupational therapy practitioners routinely provide the intervention to eligible clients. Good evidence was found that the intervention improves important outcomes and concludes that benefits substantially outweigh harm.

B—Recommend that occupational therapy practitioners routinely provide the intervention to eligible clients. At least fair evidence was found that the intervention improves important outcomes and concludes that benefits outweigh harm.

C—No recommendation is made for or against routine provision of the intervention by occupational therapy practitioners. At least fair evidence was found that the intervention can improve outcomes but concludes that the balance of the benefits and harm is too close to justify a general recommendation.

D—Recommend that occupational therapy practitioners do not provide the intervention to eligible clients. At least fair evidence was found that the intervention is ineffective or that harm outweighs benefits.

I—Insufficient evidence to recommend for or against routinely providing the intervention. Evidence that the intervention is effective is lacking, of poor quality, or conflicting and the balance of benefits and harm cannot be determined.

Buettner, 2003). Restoring occupation in the later stages of the disease in institutional settings involved examining the effectiveness of structured leisure and sensory programs to manage behavior and increase involvement (Clair & Ebberts, 1997). Social participation interventions were geared toward people in the early stages of the disease to stimulate cognition and memory while verbal skills were still intact (Brooker & Duce, 2000).

Environmental interventions were found to be effective for people in the early and middle stages of the disease using compensatory strategies such as cueing and step-by-step instructions (Graff et al., 2006). An important approach is to adjust the environmental demands to the person's abilities to avoid behavioral reactions (Swanson et al., 1994). Activity program interventions show usefulness when designed specifically to the ability level (Orsulic-Jeras et al., 2000) and arousal states (Kovach et al., 2004) of the clients. Environmental modifications can maintain or compensate for perceptual abilities that affect occupational performance. Sensory approaches such as light therapy (Skjerve, Bjorvatn, & Holsten, 2004), aromatherapy (Snow, Hovanec, & Brandt, 2004), or Snoezelen (Baillon et al., 2004) have some favorable effects on people with cognitive deficits and deserve further refinement and study. Environmental design of corridors (Elmståhl et al., 1997) and visual barriers (Dickinson et al., 1995) can positively affect orientation and exiting behaviors.

Establishing routines has been used as an intervention strategy to combat temporal impairments faced by people with dementia. Although there is no specific evidence supporting the overall use of structured routines, some advantage has been indicated for using routines for moving to a new dementia care unit (Kovach & Sterns, 1994), toileting (Doody et al., 2001), and sleeping (Alessi et al., 2005). Qualitative evidence cautions against the adherence to rigid routines for morning care for people in the later stages of the disease (Skovdahl et al., 2003) and promotion of the use of time aids (clocks, calendars) in the early stages of the disease (Nygård & Johansson, 2001).

Evidence supports modifying the activity demands by tailoring activities to the skill level of the person (Gitlin et al., 2008) and selecting activities that have personal interest to increase time on task and improve affect (Kolanowski, 2001). Occupational therapy takes the form of caregiver and staff training in activity analysis and step-by-step guidance (Dooley & Hinojosa, 2004) and compensatory approaches (Graff et al., 2006). Altering the demands and skill elicitation by providing cues, prompts, and verbal reinforcement along with other approaches improves mealtime (Watson & Green, 2006) and other ADL performance (Rogers et al., 1999).

There is much attention to prevention of falls in the elderly but little that directly targets people with Alzheimer's disease. Most studies look at falls postoperatively and, although the evidence is inconclusive, suggest that occupational therapy practitioners should participate in comprehensive programs that maintain client involvement in daily activities in hospitals (Oliver et al., 2007). Fall prevention programs work better for people with higher cognitive functioning (Jensen et al., 2003).

The evidence-based literature review provides occupational therapy practitioners with guidance in the clinical reasoning processes required to design best practice intervention planning for people with Alzheimer's disease. The therapist considers the evidence, remaining cognizant of the prioritized factors of the individual with dementia, the family supports and resources, the setting for intervention, and the pragmatic logistics of providing the services. Service delivery may be direct involvement with the person or family and caregivers, through consultation or referral with others in the health care team, or population based through program development and facility staff training. The overall goal of occupational therapy service is optimal health and well-being, meeting the occupational needs of the person with Alzheimer's disease throughout the progression of the disease.

Implications for Research

The evidence-based literature review supports the need for further and more rigorous research in institutional and home- and community-based interventions with people with Alzheimer's disease. Alzheimer's disease is a complex, multifactorial condition that affects all areas of occupation, performance patterns and skills, contexts and environments, and client factors. Its effects also resonate to the family and social group. How the disease manifests in an individual is dependent on premorbid abilities, family support and care, personality, co-morbid diagnoses, and rate of progression. The long trajectory of service over many years requires that studies accurately assess the stage and rate of cognitive decline and consider multiple factors that affect occupational performance. Just as child development investigators consider the anticipated behavioral responses on the basis of developmental age, dementia researchers must design studies for each stage of cognitive decline over the course of the disease. This process requires assessments with strong psychometric properties that measure cognitive capacity for functional performance and can serve as a standard to compare interventions across studies.

The individualized nature of occupational therapy interventions makes it a challenge to compare the interventions provided not only to individuals but also to groups. The challenge to the practitioner or researcher is to articulate the nature of service while maintaining the integrity of an individualized plan. The intervention protocols should be specific and clearly described in the literature to allow replication of the studies in different geographic areas and with diverse ethnic groups. Interventions that are setting specific—for example, home care, dementia care units, adult day services—need to provide evidence of effectiveness in one setting and be studied in alternative settings with site-specific populations. Likewise, outcomes of interventions need to be measurable and standardized to compare across studies and systematic reviews. More research is needed in establishing measurable outcomes for (a) performance in areas of occupation specific to Alzheimer's disease, (b) quality of life relative to cognitive impairment, and (c) effectiveness of interventions for caregivers.

More studies of interventions involving caregivers and family members are needed because they directly influence the health and well-being of their family member with Alzheimer's disease. Measuring outcomes of caregiver education and training programs is paramount to justify the increasing focus of service with community-based models. Research designs to evaluate a family-cen-

tered care intervention may require collaboration with family scientists in designing dyadic and small group research models. Investigating programs that meet the occupational needs of community-dwelling people with Alzheimer's disease must include the well-being of caregivers and other family members affected by the disease.

Investigations of occupational performance of people with Alzheimer's disease demand a team approach. Because of the indeterminate method for diagnosis, medical experts must align with other disciplines to gather information for a consensus diagnosis. Studies of this population require an understanding of the types of dementia to narrow the subject pool to those with a definitive diagnosis. Other dementia-related disorders can mask or augment symptoms of the disease and affect occupational performance beyond the limitations that stem from cognitive decline. A team approach to research reflects the team approach to care. Collaboration also should involve dementia care experts in the field who can generate the pressing and pertinent questions to be studied and participate in collecting data and developing interventions.

Implications for Education

Implications for education are threefold: (1) increased understanding of neuroscience and neurorehabilitation, (2) knowledge of family science and family-centered care models of intervention, and (3) community-based program development and evaluation. Occupational therapy curricula should enhance the basic understanding of cognitive processes, including memory, executive function, attention and concentration, language, and perception. Appropriate training in the selection, administration, and interpretation of assessment tools for dementia-related conditions is vital. With more sophisticated and specialized practice areas growing, curricular decisions should be made on the basis of the most pressing health care needs of the populations that occupational therapy practitioners serve. With the increasing prevalence of Alzheimer's disease, this training potentially can affect hospital, outpatient, skilled nursing, transitional and subacute, home, and community-based care provision.

The evidence is strong that interventions that consider a family-centered or caregiver-focused approach to intervention are more successful than a direct service approach with the client. Occupational therapy curricula should include content in family theory and family science that can train future therapists in designing intervention approaches beyond direct service to the individual. This curricula may include honing family interview and observation skills; conducting family meetings; developing skills for facilitating family decision making; and knowing policies, including privacy protection of confidential health-related information. Occupational therapy graduates should have confidence in working with families and caregivers in the spectrum of settings where people with Alzheimer's are served.

Education also must emphasize skill development in community-based intervention planning for the occupational therapy student. Program development and evaluation, currently a standard for occupational therapy education, could be enhanced with public engagement opportunities with this population. Designing, implementing, and evaluating activity programs in facilities that serve elders in memory care are valuable and effective learning experiences.

Implications for Practice

The key to effective intervention planning is accurate and standardized assessment of occupational performance. Occupational therapy practitioners should have the skills to administer the assessments and, for occupational therapists, the clinical reasoning skills to consider multiple sources of information that contribute to the intervention plan. Interventions must be selected on the basis of evidence that it has been shown to be effective and implemented in a conscientious manner to produce measurable results. For interventions designed for people with Alzheimer's disease, studies have shown that the focus on the context and environment are effective rather than restorative treatment for the individual. Interventions that provide services in the community, in the natural environment, using objects familiar to the person are more effective than a clinical, unfamiliar

setting. Providing caregiver training in new approaches to assisting the client promotes increased engagement in daily living skills and reduced caregiver burden more than client skill training. Individualized activities that meet clients' ability levels encourage more involvement than general activity programs designed for groups. Interventions must be designed considering the stage of the disease, and practitioners need to be flexible around those transition points. For instance, assistive devices may be useful in the early stages of the disease and not used or improperly used in the later stages of the disease. Likewise, structured routines may benefit temporal organization in the early to middle stages of the disease, whereas greater flexibility with routine is important in the later stages of the disease.

For each client, the practitioner must consider the multiple factors that affect occupational performance to meet the client's needs in the context of his or her living environment and resources available. The evidence supports a broad set of skills and knowledge of practical and applicable strategies to tailor the interventions to the person. At the same time, it requires creativity, adaptability, and persistence on the part of the therapist to find solutions to evolving problems that arise in the care of the client with dementia. With the gradual changes that occur over years, the services should be provided at intervals throughout the course of the disease and target both the immediate needs and short- and long-term planning for future needs.

In summary, occupational therapy has a distinct role in contributing toward the health and well-being for people with Alzheimer's disease—a role that is supported by evidence. There is a need for specialized and experienced therapists in this area of practice that parallels the increasing number of people diagnosed annually with the disease. The intervention planning is complex, dynamic over time, and involves groups of people beyond the client with the disease. Occupational therapy practice with this population requires ongoing innovations in service delivery, expanded teaching and learning opportunities in education to prepare practitioners for this area of practice, and collaboration with researchers to ensure evidence to support best practice.

Appendix A.
Preparation and Qualifications of Occupational Therapists and Occupational Therapy Assistants

Who Are Occupational Therapists?

To practice as an occupational therapist, the individual trained in the United States

- Has graduated from an occupational therapy program accredited by the Accreditation Council for Occupational Therapy Education (ACOTE®) or predecessor organizations;
- Has successfully completed a period of supervised fieldwork experience required by the recognized educational institution where the applicant met the academic requirements of an educational program for occupational therapists that is accredited by ACOTE or predecessor organizations;
- Has passed a nationally recognized entry-level examination for occupational therapists; and
- Fulfills state requirements for licensure, certification, or registration.

Educational Programs for the Occupational Therapist

These include the following:
- Biological, physical, social, and behavioral sciences
- Basic tenets of occupational therapy
- Occupational therapy theoretical perspectives
- Screening and evaluation
- Formulation and implementation of an intervention plan
- Context of service delivery
- Management of occupational therapy services (master's level)

- Leadership and management (doctoral level)
- Use of research
- Professional ethics, values, and responsibilities.

The fieldwork component of the program is designed to develop competent, entry-level, generalist occupational therapists by providing experience with a variety of clients across the life span and in a variety of settings. Fieldwork is integral to the program's curriculum design and includes an in-depth experience in delivering occupational therapy services to clients, focusing on the application of purposeful and meaningful occupation and/or research, administration, and management of occupational therapy services. The fieldwork experience is designed to promote clinical reasoning and reflective practice, to transmit the values and beliefs that enable ethical practice, and to develop professionalism and competence in career responsibilities. Doctoral-level students also must complete a doctoral experiential component designed to develop advanced skills beyond a generalist level.

Who Are Occupational Therapy Assistants?

To practice as an occupational therapy assistant, the individual trained in the United States
- Has graduated from an occupational therapy assistant program accredited by ACOTE or predecessor organizations;
- Has successfully completed a period of supervised fieldwork experience required by the recognized

educational institution where the applicant met the academic requirements of an educational program for occupational therapy assistants that is accredited by ACOTE or predecessor organizations;

- Has passed a nationally recognized entry-level examination for occupational therapy assistants; and
- Fulfills state requirements for licensure, certification, or registration.

Educational Programs for the Occupational Therapy Assistant

These include the following:
- Biological, physical, social, and behavioral sciences
- Basic tenets of occupational therapy
- Screening and assessment
- Intervention and implementation
- Context of service delivery
- Assistance in management of occupational therapy services
- Professional literature
- Professional ethics, values, and responsibilities.

The fieldwork component of the program is designed to develop competent, entry-level, generalist occupational therapy assistants by providing experience with a variety of clients across the life span and in a variety of settings. Fieldwork is integral to the program's curriculum design and includes an in-depth experience in delivering occupational therapy services to clients, focusing on the application of purposeful and meaningful occupation. The fieldwork experience is designed to promote clinical reasoning appropriate to the occupational therapy assistant role, to transmit the values and beliefs that enable ethical practice, and to develop professionalism and competence in career responsibilities.

Regulation of Occupational Therapy Practice

All occupational therapists and occupational therapy assistants must practice under federal and state law. Currently, 50 states, the District of Columbia, Puerto Rico, and Guam have enacted laws regulating the practice of occupational therapy.

Note. The majority of this information is taken from the *Accreditation Standards for a Doctoral-Degree-Level Educational Program for the Occupational Therapist* (ACOTE, 2007a), *Accreditation Standards for a Master's-Degree-Level Educational Program for the Occupational Therapist* (ACOTE, 2007b), and *Accreditation Standards for an Educational Program for the Occupational Therapy Assistant* (ACOTE, 2007c).

■ ■ ■

Appendix B.
Selected *CPT*™ Coding for Occupational Therapy Evaluations and Interventions

The following chart is a guide to assist in making clinically appropriate decisions in selecting the most relevant *CPT* code to describe occupation therapy evaluation and intervention. Occupational therapy practitioners should use the most appropriate code from the current *CPT* based on specific services provided, individual patient goals, payer policy, and common usage.

Examples of Occupational Therapy Evaluation and Intervention	Suggested *CPT*™ Code(s)
• Individual 1:1 functional evaluation using standardized and nonstandardized assessments • Bill total time for evaluation • Bill one evaluation per episode of care	**97003—Occupational Therapy Evaluation** Initial evaluation of performance in areas of occupation, performance skills, performance patterns, context and environment, activity demands, and client factors
• Individual 1:1 functional evaluation after initial evaluation using standardized and nonstandardized assessments • Bill total time for reevaluation • Updated plan of care required	**97004—Occupational Therapy Reevaluation** Formal reevaluation of performance due to change of status, change in diagnosis, or when care plan requires significant revisions

• Qualified health professional time for administration and interpretation of standardized cognitive assessments and preparation of the report
• Time billed per hour of service. An occupational therapy initial evaluation must precede cognitive testing. Cognitive assessments may include
  – Cognitive Performance Test
  – Executive Function Test
  – Cognistat
  – CMT
  – LOTCA
	96125—Standardized Cognitive Performance Testing
	Evaluation of neurocognition, including global cognitive functions, executive function, memory, learning, problem solving, constructional praxis, language, attention, and other neural substrates for occupational performance

• Direct 1:1 assistive technology assessment to restore, augment, or compensate for existing function, optimize functional tasks, or maximize environmental accessibility • An occupational therapy initial evaluation must precede an assistive technology assessment • Time billed in 15-min increments Note: Training in the use of the AT device can be billed under the code for self-care/home management training (97535).	**97755—Assistive Technology Assessment** Assessment of the client's need for advanced assistive technology to adapt seating systems and environmental controls to compensate for cognitive loss and minimize mobility restrictions (e.g., exiting alarms, first alert systems, motion detectors) **92605 & 92607** Augmentative and alternative communication devices

(continued)

Examples of Occupational Therapy Evaluation and Intervention	Suggested *CPT*™ Code(s)
• Direct 1:1 training for persons in early stages of the disease who can benefit from new learning; document cognitive skills and compensatory strategies • Time billed in 15 minute increments	**97532—Development of Cognitive Skills** Intervene through training in the use of memory aids (calendars, lists, timers), organizers (schedules, structured routines), problem solving (emergency contact processes such as phone speed dial), and other compensatory strategies (photo phones, family monitoring, medication management systems)
• Direct 1:1 training for persons and/or caregivers in compensatory and safety procedures, including designing, fabricating, modifying, and training in assistive devices and adaptive equipment related to ADL goal	**97535—Self-Care/Home Management/ADL Training** Intervene through training in self-care or ADLs, IADLs, including meal preparation and safety procedures
• Direct 1:1 application of neurorehabilitation techniques to facilitate motor and sensory processing and promote adaptive responses to sitting, standing, and posturing with the goal of improved safety in daily activity; time billed in 15-min increments	**97112—Therapeutic Procedure** Intervene through modulation (facilitation and inhibition) of sensory input and stimulation of motor responses (movement, balance, coordination, kinesthetic, posture, or proprioceptive) using neuromuscular reeducation and neurorehabilitation approaches
• Direct 1:1 individualized exercise program for physical skill development and instruction and training in a home exercise program • Time billed in 15-min increments	**97110—Therapeutic Exercise** Intervene to restore client factors including strength, endurance, flexibility, and active, assistive, and passive range of motion using exercises such as progressive resistive, prolonged stretch, or isokinetic, isotonic, or isometric strengthening, or closed kinetic chain
• Direct 1:1 individualized therapeutic activities or use of an activity as an intervention, related to performance of specific functional tasks • Time billed in 15-min increments	**97530—Therapeutic Activities** Intervene to restore functional performance in areas of occupation including ADLs (transfer to bed or toilet), IADLs (lifting pan from stove), work (cleaning floor), leisure, or social participation (balancing with partner in social dancing)
• Direct group activities for 2 to 4 clients who engage in the same activity to support a common goal • Document number of clients in group and total time for each client in the group • Code is billed as 1 unit for each client	**97150—Group Therapeutic Procedure** Intervene in group setting using therapeutic exercise (seated yoga for flexibility) or functional activities (energy conservation for chronic fatigue) with clients with similar goals
• Direct participation in a formal medical team conference (not rounds) for clients (with or without client and family present) with chronic or multiple health conditions • Conference must be 30 minutes or greater and is reported as 1 unit • One provider per specialty may bill per conference	**99366*** Patient and/or family present **99368*** Patient and/or family not present **Medical Team Conference ≥30 minutes** Conference with interdisciplinary health care team to report evaluation findings (within 60 days of evaluation) and provide recommendations contributing to the formulation or review of a comprehensive care plan

Note. Document client and/or family response to intervention and demonstration or verbalization of skills learned. Clearly document evaluations, assessments, and interventions as distinct time periods if billed in the same session; use *CPT* code language, e.g. "Self-Care/Home Management Training included compensatory strategies in selection of clothing" and "Cognitive Skill training included signage reminders to use appropriate outer ware."

Medical team conferences are not billable to Medicare; however, these codes may be useful for reporting productivity.

Note. CMT = Contextual Memory Test; LOTCA = Lowenstein Occupational Therapy Cognitive Assessment; AT = assistive technology; ADLs = activities of daily living; IADLs = instrumental activities of daily living.

The *CPT 2010* codes referenced in this document do not represent all of the possible codes that may be used in occupational therapy evaluation and intervention. Not all payers will reimburse for all codes. Refer to *CPT 2010* for the complete list of available codes.

CPT™ is a trademark of the American Medical Association (AMA). *CPT* five-digit codes, nomenclature, and other data are copyright 2010 by the American Medical Association. All Rights Reserved. Reprinted with permission. No fee schedules, basic units, relative values, or related listings are included in *CPT*. The AMA assumes no liability for the data contained herein.

Codes shown refer to *CPT 2010. CPT* codes are updated annually. New and revised codes become effective January 1. Always refer to annual updated *CPT* publication for most current codes.

Appendix C.
2009 Selected *ICD-9-CM* Codes

Alzheimer's disease	331.0
Disease or sclerosis	331.0
With dementia with behavioral disturbance	331.0 [294.11]
With dementia without behavioral disturbance	331.0 [294.10]
Atrophy brain progressive	331.9
Brain general lobular	341.9
Dementias	290.0
Senile dementia uncomplicated	290.0
Presenile dementia	290.1
Senile dementia with delusional or depressive symptoms	290.2
Senile dementia with delirium	290.3
Vascular dementia	290.4
Other specified senile psychotic conditions	290.8
Unspecified senile psychotic condition	290.9
Alcoholic psychoses	291
Delirium tremens	291.0
Drug psychoses	292
Transient organic psychotic conditions	293
Delirium	293.0
Other organic psychotic conditions (chronic)	294
Amnestic disorder in conditions classified elsewhere	294.0
Dementia in conditions classified elsewhere	294.1
Other persistent mental disorders due to conditions classified elsewhere	294.8
Unspecified persistent mental disorders due to conditions classified elsewhere	294.9

Note. Other *ICD-9* codes may be used in occupational therapy practice. For additional coding information, see www.cms.hhs.gov/ICD9ProviderDiagnosticCodes.

■ ■ ■

Appendix D.
Evidence-Based Practice

One of the greatest challenges facing health care systems, service providers, public education, and policymakers is to ensure that scarce resources are used efficiently. The growing interest in outcomes research and evidence-based health care over the past 30 years, and the more recent interest in evidence-based education can in part be explained by these system-level challenges in the United States and internationally. In response to the demands of the cost-oriented health care system in which occupational therapy practice is often embedded, occupational therapists and occupational therapy assistants are routinely asked to justify the value of the services they provide on the basis of the scientific evidence. The scientific literature provides an important source of legitimacy and authority for demonstrating the value of health care and education services. Thus, occupational therapists, other health care practitioners, and educators are increasingly called on to use the literature to inform their practice and to demonstrate the value of the interventions and instruction they provide to clients and students.

What Is an Evidence-Based Practice Perspective?

According to Law and Baum (1998), *evidence-based occupational therapy practice* "uses research evidence together with clinical knowledge and reasoning to make decisions about interventions that are effective for a specific client" (p. 131). An evidence-based perspective is based on the assumption that scientific evidence of the effectiveness of occupational therapy intervention can be judged to be more or less strong and valid according to a hierarchy of research designs

or an assessment of the quality of the research. AOTA uses standards of evidence modeled from standards developed in evidence-based medicine. This model standardizes and ranks the value of scientific evidence for biomedical practice using the grading system shown in Table D1. In this system, the highest levels of evidence include systematic reviews of the literature, meta-analyses, and randomized controlled trials. In randomized controlled trials, the outcomes of an intervention are compared with the outcomes of a control group, and participation in either group is allocated randomly. The evidence-based literature review presented here includes *Level I* randomized controlled trials; *Level II* studies, in which assignment to a treatment or a control group is not randomized (cohort study); *Level III* studies, which do not have a control group; *Level IV* studies, which are single-case experimental design, sometimes reported over several participants; and *Level V* studies, which are case reports and expert opinion that include narrative literature reviews and consensus statements. In addition, qualitative studies were included in two of the focused question reviews. The inclusion of the qualitative literature provides additional information in areas of limited research.

This study was initiated and supported by the AOTA as part of the Evidence-Based Literature Review project.

Seven focused questions were developed for the evidence-based literature review of occupational therapy interventions for adults with Alzheimer's disease. The questions were generated in conjunction with a group of content experts in Alzheimer's disease and evidence-based practice. They were developed and reviewed to provide needed information to update the previously

Table D1. Levels of Evidence for Occupational Therapy Outcomes Research

Levels of Evidence	Definitions
Level I	Systematic reviews, meta-analyses, randomized controlled trials
Level II	Two groups, nonrandomized studies (e.g., cohort, case-control)
Level III	One group, nonrandomized (e.g., before and after, pretest and posttest)
Level IV	Descriptive studies that include analysis of outcomes (e.g., single-subject design, case series)
Level V	Case reports and expert opinion that include narrative literature reviews and consensus statements

Note. From "Evidence-based medicine: What it is and what it isn't," by D. L. Sackett, W. M. Rosenberg, J. A. Muir Gray, R. B. Haynes, & W. S. Richardson, 1996, *British Medical Journal, 312*, 71–72. Copyright © 1996 by the *British Medical Journal*. Adapted with permission.

published guidelines for the practice of occupational therapy for adults with Alzheimer's disease.

The following focused questions were included in the review:

1. What is the evidence for the effect of interventions designed to establish, modify, and maintain activities of daily living (ADLs), instrumental activities of daily living (IADLs), leisure, and social participation on the quality of life, health and wellness, and client and caregiver satisfaction for persons with dementia? (Areas of Occupation)
2. What is the evidence for the effect of interventions designed to modify and maintain perceptual abilities on the occupational performance of people with dementia? (Perception)
3. What is the evidence for the effectiveness of interventions designed to establish, modify, or maintain routines on the occupational performance, quality of life, health and wellness, and client and caregiver satisfaction of people with Alzheimer's disease? (Routines)
4. What is the effect of environmental-based interventions (e.g., Montessori and Snoezelen) on performance, affect, and behavior in both the home and institutions for people with Alzheimer's disease? (Environment)
5. What is the effectiveness of interventions designed to modify the activity demands of the occupations of self-care, work, leisure, and social participation for people with Alzheimer's disease? (Activity Demands)

6. What is the evidence for the effect of interventions to prevent falls in people with dementia? (Fall Prevention)
7. What is the effectiveness of educational and supportive strategies for caregivers of people with dementia on the ability to maintain the participation in that role? (Caregiver Strategies)

Inclusion and exclusion criteria are critical to the systematic review process because they provide the structure for the quality, type, and years of publication of the literature incorporated into a review. The review of all seven questions was limited to the peer-review scientific literature published in English. The review also included consolidated information sources such as the Cochrane Collaboration. Except as described here, the literature included in the review was published since 1987, with the study populations including participants with dementia or their caregivers. The review excluded data from presentations, conference proceedings, non–peer-reviewed research literature, research reports, dissertations, and theses.

One team headed by Lori Letts, PhD, OT Reg. (Ont.), of McMaster University, Hamilton, Ontario, reviewed intervention questions focusing on areas of occupation, perception, and routines. These reviews included literature published between 1994 and 2005. The areas of occupation review included interventions that focused on at least one of the following: ADLs, IADLs, leisure, or social participation. Studies were considered for the review if they included at least one of the following outcome measures: quality of life, health, wellness, and client or caregiver satisfaction. Articles with study samples of people with AIDS-related dementia were excluded from the review. The perception review included studies that described and evaluated interventions that targeted perception, either improving or maintaining perception, or using remaining perceptual abilities. In addition, studies included in the perception review reported functional or occupational performance outcomes. The routines review included studies that described an intervention on the basis of the use of routine, described responses to the use of routine in the course of daily care, or described interactions during routines. Studies were excluded from the review if there was no report of data or systematic observations of the outcomes of the use of routines. For all three reviews, the following databases were searched: AgeLine, CINAHL, Medline, PsycInfo, EMBASE, and HealthSTAR. In addition, the Cochrane Library, OT Seeker, and Allied and Complementary Medicine were searched for the perception and routines questions. Bibliographies of selected studies in all three reviews were hand searched to locate additional potential articles. Team members developed the search strategies, and a research librarian with a specialty in rehabilitation science was consulted to finalize the search strategy. Table D2 presents the search strategies for all three reviews. A team member conducted the searches, and review members discussed

the search results to ensure that key articles or areas of research had not been overlooked and that articles met the inclusion criteria. Group consensus was used to resolve any uncertainties. For the review focusing on areas of occupation, 6,621 titles and abstracts were reviewed, and 291 articles were reviewed in full. Twenty-six articles fulfilled the inclusion and exclusion criteria for the review. A total of 3,766 titles and abstracts were reviewed from the perception search, and 111 of those articles were retrieved. Twenty-eight articles were included in the final review. For the review focusing on routines, 823 titles and abstracts were reviewed, and 24 articles were retrieved. Fourteen articles were included in the routines review.

The second team, led by Rene Padilla, PhD, OTR, FAOTA, with doctoral students in the occupational therapy program at Creighton University, Omaha, Nebraska, conducted the reviews on the environment, activity demands, fall prevention, and caregiver strategies. All reviews were completed in 2007 with the exception of the review on caregiver strategies, which was completed in 2008. Participants of the included studies were people with dementia, except for the falls and caregiver strategies, which focused on the caregivers. Interventions included in all reviews were specific to the question (e.g., interventions for activity demands related to self-care and other ADLs, IADLs, work, leisure, or social participation) and fit within the

Table D2. Search Strategy for Systematic Reviews on Areas of Occupation, Perception, and Routines

Category	Key Search Terms
Patient/Client Population	Dementia (exploded) key word and text word
Intervention—Areas of Occupation	(ADLs) OR (IADLs or household or household management) OR (social interaction or social participation or social behavior or interpersonal interaction or interpersonal interactions or participation or social behavior or religion or religious practice or worship) OR (recreation or leisure or leisure participation) OR (sexual behavior or sexual intimacy or intimacy)
Intervention—Perception	Perception, perceptual abilities or perceptual impairment (including searching for the terms: perceptual discrimination, apraxia, agnosia, stereognosis, spatial discrimination, spatial relations, depth perception, color perception, visuospatial impairment, hemianopsia, hemianopia, way finding, body awareness, body image, body scheme, auditory priming, auditory perception, left right discrimination, speech perception, visual perception, sensory integration)
Intervention—Routines	Activity patterns OR schedules OR routine OR habit OR habits
Comparison	Not included in search strategy
Outcomes	Not included in search strategy

scope of practice of occupational therapy practitioners. This set of reviews included Level I, II, and III studies, except for the environment review, which included a Level IV study. For all reviews, the following databases were searched: Medline, OT Search, AgeLine, CINAHL, PsycInfo, Google Scholar, Academic Search Premiere, Science Direct, and Web of Science. In addition, the Cochrane Library was searched for the falls and caregiver strategies reviews. Dr. Padilla developed the search strategies, and a medical librarian, AOTA staff, and a consultant to the AOTA Evidence-Based Practice Project reviewed them. Table D3 presents the search strategies for the four questions reviewed by the Creighton team. After graduation of the doctoral students, Dr. Padilla performed additional searching to update the reviews. A total of 17,000 abstracts were reviewed for the four-question search, and 127 articles were reviewed in depth. From those, 62 articles met the inclusion and exclusion criteria for final selection.

Table D4 presents the number of studies included in the complete review, included in each focused question, as well as the composition of the articles included in the review by level of evidence. The two teams working on each focused question reviewed the articles according to their quality (scientific rigor and lack of bias) and levels of evidence. Each article included in the review was then abstracted using an evidence table that provides a summary of the methods and findings of the article, an appraisal of the strengths and weaknesses of the study on the basis of the design, methodology, and implications for occupational therapy. Review authors also completed a Critically Appraised Topic (CAT), a summary and appraisal of the key findings, clinical bottom line, and implica-

Table D3. Search Strategy for Systematic Reviews on Environmental Interventions, Activity Demands, Falls, and Caregiver Interventions

Review Question	Category	Key Search Terms
Environmental Interventions	Patient/Client Population	Alzheimer's, dementia
	Intervention	Strategy, technique, treatment, intervention, environment, Montessori, Snoezelen, Environmental Skill-Building Program (ESP), progressively lowered stress threshold, multisensory, aromatherapy, bright light therapy
	Outcome	Self-care, ADLs, work, employment, occupation, vocation, job, leisure, recreation, socialization, interaction, social participation, communication, social interaction, social engagement, engagement, affect, emotion, agitation, behavior
Activity Demands	Patient/Client Population	Alzheimer's, dementia
	Intervention	Strategy, technique, treatment, intervention, adapt, modify, adjust, change, alter
	Outcome	Self-care, ADLs, work, employment, occupation, vocation, job, leisure, recreation, socialization, interaction, social participation, communication, social interaction, social engagement, engagement
Falls	Patient/Client Population	Alzheimer's, dementia, cognitive impairment, elderly
	Intervention	Fall prevention, intervention, safety
	Outcome	Fall reduction, fall prevention, injury reduction
Caregiver Interventions	Patient/Client Population	Caregivers, careers, helpers, family, Alzheimer's, dementia
	Intervention	Education, psychoeducation, intervention, support, strategy
	Outcome	Depression, mental health, burden, longevity, knowledge
	Comparison	Not included in search strategy for review questions

Table D4. Number and Levels of Evidence for Articles Included in Each Review Question

Review Question	Number of Articles Included in Review						Total in Each Review
	Level I	Level II	Level III	Level IV	Level V	Qualitative	
Areas of Occupation	7	1	11	7	0	0	26
Perception	10	4	8	5	0	1	28
Routines	7	0	1	0	1	5	14
Environmental Interventions	13	6	2	1	0	0	21
Activity Demands	6	0	1	0	0	0	7
Falls	3	0	2	0	0	0	5
Caregiver Interventions	23	1	4	0	0	0	28
Total for Each Level	69	12	29	13	1	6	
						Total in All Reviews	129

tions for occupational therapy of the articles included in the review for each question. Review authors also completed Critically Appraised Papers for all articles included in the perception and routines reviews and the Level I, II, and III articles for the occupation review. AOTA staff and the Evidence-Based Practice Project consultant reviewed the evidence tables and CATs to ensure quality control.

Limitations of selected studies incorporated in the review include small sample size, lack of power analysis, and limited detail regarding recruitment of participants. In several cases, the study group was heterogeneous and may not have been representative of the population with dementia. Depending on the level of evidence, there may have been a lack of randomization, lack of control group, and limited statistical reporting. In many cases, the studies included both a limited description of the outcome measure and explanation of the psychometric properties of the measures. In some cases, the outcome measures were subjective, and there was limited follow-up of the intervention. It is difficult to separate the effects of a single intervention that is part of a multimodal intervention. In addition, adverse effects of an intervention may not have been included, and some studies did not control for confounders in the analysis. Several of the qualitative studies were limited by the amount of information provided about the data collection and analytic procedures. Because several were published before 2001, the review author indicated that this may be a reflection of fewer demands related to trustworthiness and credibility as part of a general limited understanding of qualitative research in older literature.

■ ■ ■

Appendix E.
Evidence Tables

EVIDENCE TABLE: What is the evidence for the effect of interventions designed to establish, modify, and maintain activities of daily living (ADLs), instrumental activities of daily living (IADLs), leisure, and social participation on the quality of life, health and wellness, and client and caregiver satisfaction for persons with dementia?

Author/Year	Study Objectives	Level/Design/ Participants	Intervention and Outcome Measures	Results	Study Limitations	Implications for Occupational Therapy
Activities of daily living (ADLs)						
Altus, Engelman, & Mathews, 2002	The objective was to examine the effect of using serving dishes (family-style meals) versus prepared plates on participation in mealtime tasks by residents with dementia who still possess independent eating skills. The authors hypothesized that the use of family-style meals would result in an increase in independent resident behavior and an increase in appropriate communication.	Level IV ABAB reversal Participants Convenience sample, $n = 6$ residents living in a locked dementia unit. 1 resident died before study completion. 5 reported participants were women; mean age = 80. Diagnosis was dementia or AD, moderate to severe (MMSE = mean 8/30). All participants were ambulatory and able to eat meals independently or with minimal assistance from the nursing assistant.	Intervention ■ Prepared plates changed to serving dishes (family style) ■ Praise from CNA Outcome Measures ■ Observations (3×/wk lasting a mean of 87 min) of participation using a category checklist and accounting for level of assistance ■ Communication of inappropriate versus appropriate using interval recording ■ Praise tally	Participation at baseline had a mean of 10%. Family-style meals were associated with an increase to 24% mean. Family-style meals plus training of a CNA in offering praise and graduated prompting were associated with an increase in the mean to 64% participation. Communication levels rose similarly, but less dramatically, from 5.5% to 10.6% to 17.9% respectively (all reported as means).	This study began as an ABA design, but when limited gains were noted, the authors added an additional B condition (CNA training), which resulted in a dramatic increase in participation. There was no condition of prepared plates plus trained CNA interaction, which may be the most important variable. Small sample size and limited generalizability were limitations in this study.	Although there are limitations, there is an opportunity here for occupational therapists to provide training to support staff on graded assistance during mealtimes and educate on the use of positive reinforcement, as the trained CNAs' interactions appeared to be a pivotal point (again, this was not thoroughly tested) in increased interaction. It supports the need to prevent excess disability in people with dementia and to reinforce the use of remaining abilities. Of note, the CNA reported family-style meals were more satisfying and actually less work than prepared plates.

Altus, D. E., Engelman, K. K., & Mathews, R. M. (2002). Using family-style meals to increase participation and communication in persons with dementia. *Journal of Gerontological Nursing, 28,* 47–53.

(continued)

EVIDENCE TABLE: What is the evidence for the effect of interventions designed to establish, modify, and maintain activities of daily living (ADLs), instrumental activities of daily living (IADLs), leisure, and social participation on the quality of life, health and wellness, and client and caregiver satisfaction for persons with dementia? *(continued)*

Author/Year	Study Objectives	Level/Design/ Participants	Intervention and Outcome Measures	Results	Study Limitations	Implications for Occupational Therapy
Beattie, Algase, & Song, 2004	The objective was to determine the effect of the systematic use of a behavioral nursing intervention on mealtime behavior of wanderers. The authors hypothesized that systematic behavioral intervention during a 20-min mealtime would ■ Increase the total time spent seated ■ Decrease the frequency of table leaving events ■ Increase the proportion of food and fluid consumed over baseline levels of food consumption ■ Promote weight change in a favorable direction for those who have less than ideal body weight	<u>Level III</u> Before and after <u>Participants</u> 3 dementia unit residents (2 women, 1 man) with probable AD and identified as wanderers or table leavers and without competing explanations for the wandering. They had been residents for approximately 2 yr. Study documents further similarities.	<u>Intervention</u> Systematic reinforcement of sitting-at-table behavior used communication strategies of conversation about the meal, eating or the mealtime experience, and specific social behavior, such as smiling. Systematic stopping of table-leaving behavior was also used as needed. Intervention was conducted for each resident individually for a 5-week period with 2 repeats of the intervention. During the intervention week, each resident received the intervention daily for 5 days in the first 20 min of the mealtime. <u>Outcome Measures</u> ■ Frequency and duration of table leaving (tally) ■ Weight of food eaten, proportion of food and fluid accepted ■ Body weight measured 3×/wk	Within case independent *t*-tests All 3 participants showed statistically significant increases of time sitting at the table ($p = .014$, $p = .001$, $p = .032$), 2 of 3 participants showed a statistically significant decrease in table leaving ($p = .0005$, $p = .0009$, $p = .060$). 2 of 3 participants showed a statistically significant increase in food intake ($p = .969$, $p = .000$, $p = .000$). Intake of fluids did not change. No significant difference in body weight occurred; however, there was evidence of weight maintenance during the study. This finding may be clinically significant because all participants were on a weight loss trajectory before the study.	Small sample size, nonrandomized mealtime intervention schedule (time of day affects agitation) BMI would be a more meaningful measure than weight alone.	Stability of weight is a clinically important outcome in dementia, especially for residents at increased risk for weight loss due to wandering away during meals. Occupational therapists can be involved with the mealtime experience with emphasis on the occupation of eating by assessing and facilitating remaining abilities. Individual interventions might be recommended to address multiple factors (environmental, physical, cognitive). The occupational therapist's role is to develop the intervention strategies that fit within the parameters of nursing resources, and to provide education to enable staff to implement these strategies on a daily basis.

Beattie, E. R., Algase, D. L., & Song, J. (2004). Keeping wandering nursing home residents at the table: Improving food intake using a behavioral communication intervention. *Aging and Mental Health, 8,* 109–116.

| Boylston, Ryan, Brown, & Westfall, 1995 | The study objective was to determine whether or not there were correlations between changes in diet (food texture) to maintain oral intake and decreases in functioning. | <u>Level III</u>
The authors describe this as a retrospective study; however, data appear to have been collected prospectively and then extracted through chart review.

<u>Participants</u>
14 participants with a mean age of 83.9 (*SD* 6.8).

3 men and 11 women participated. Participants attended a day care center where medical and rehabilitation are provided. All participants were certified for nursing home placement. | Intervention for this study consisted of the eating and swallowing evaluation and implementation of the food texture recommendation of the speech pathologist.

<u>Outcome Measures</u>
■ MMSE
■ ADLs (simple counts of ADL dependencies)
■ IADLs (no detail provided re: how IADL were measured)
■ Weight
■ Diet texture (ordinal)
  – Puree
  – Mechanical soft with ground meat
  – Soft
  – Regular texture | Regression analysis was used to assess the relationship between ADLs, IADLs, diet order, and weight. However, it is unclear whether diet texture was always the dependent variable.

After the intervention, a significant difference was found ($p = .0033$) between the IADLs and diet. As a decline in function occurred, patients who had changes in diet texture (down the scale from regular to puree) experienced increased food intake determined by the maintenance of body weight.

A trend was found ($p = .18892$) between diet and weight.

No interactions between ADLs, IADLs, weight, and diet were found to be significant. | Limited sample size and low level of evidence make generalization difficult. Regression analyses are not clearly presented, making interpretation difficult.

Limited information is provided about how the participants were recruited and the inclusion/exclusion criteria, resulting in the possibility of selection bias. | Weight can be considered an indicator of health. This study suggests that when people show a behavioral intolerance for food texture, softening the diet can increase intake and result in maintaining weight. However, therapists need to conduct a comprehensive assessment to establish whether food texture is influencing intake.

The authors note that a physical assessment of eating and swallowing should always be conducted to rule out aspiration risks. |

Boylston, E., Ryan, C., Brown, C., & Westfall, B. (1995). Increasing oral intake in dementia patients by altering food texture. *American Journal of Alzheimer's Disease, 10*, 37–39.

(continued)

EVIDENCE TABLE: What is the evidence for the effect of interventions designed to establish, modify, and maintain activities of daily living (ADLs), instrumental activities of daily living (IADLs), leisure, and social participation on the quality of life, health and wellness, and client and caregiver satisfaction for persons with dementia? *(continued)*

Author/Year	Study Objectives	Level/Design/ Participants	Intervention and Outcome Measures	Results	Study Limitations	Implications for Occupational Therapy
Nochajski, Tomita, & Mann, 1996	Study identified 3 specific research questions: ■ What are the reasons for dissatisfaction with assistive devices by persons with cognitive impairments and their care providers? ■ Will training on the use of assistive devices and environmental interventions and professional support promote participant and care provider acceptance of and satisfaction with assistive devices? ■ Will the use of assistive devices help maintain the functional abilities of persons with cognitive impairments?	<u>Level III</u> 1 group, pre–post study Inclusion criteria: Mental Status Exam score between 10 and 23. Mean = 15.7 *Exclusion:* Participants whose MMSE score appeared influenced by language or literacy were not included in the study. *N* = 20 (10 women, 10 men) Mean age = 79.0 90% White 65% high school education 50% widowed 80% lived with someone	<u>Intervention</u> Assistive devices and environmental interventions were provided or existing devices were adapted to meet specific needs. Participants and care providers were trained on the devices, including supervised practice. Telephone support was provided at 2-week, 4-week, 2-month, 4-month, and 6-month intervals. <u>Outcome Measures</u> ■ MMSE ■ FIM™ ■ Multidimensional Functional Assessment of Older Adults (OARS) ■ Care Provider Burden Scale ■ Environmental Survey ■ Activity Performance Worksheet ■ Assistive Device User Survey	*Research Question 1:* ■ Greater satisfaction was reported for cognitive devices. ■ 68% of cognitive devices were used compared with 48% of the physical devices ■ Primary reason for dissatisfaction was the limited cognitive abilities of the individual *Research Question 2:* Participants with higher MMSE scores (15–23) and their caregivers were significantly more likely to accept physical ($\chi^2 = 8.78$; $p < .005$) and cognitive ($\chi^2 = 5.66$; $p = .015$) devices than participants with low MMSE scores. Significant difference in satisfaction for physical devices from preintervention to postintervention ($\chi^2 = 5.97$; $p = .015$). No significant difference for cognitive devices.	Data on the effectiveness of assistive devices in maintaining functional abilities were not presented. The third research question is answered through presentation of 4 clinical scenarios. The authors report the Assistive Device User Survey needs to be refined to improve internal consistency of the second and third factors and test–retest and intra- and interrater reliability also need to be established.	Results of this study support the use of skilled professionals (occupational therapists) in providing the proper training on physical assistive devices to attempt to increase the user satisfaction. Future research is still needed to determine the effectiveness of professional intervention related to maintaining function through assistive devices for persons with cognitive impairment.

Nochajski, S. M., Tomita, M. R., & Mann, W. C. (1996). The use and satisfaction with assistive devices by older persons with cognitive impairments: A pilot intervention study. *Topics in Geriatric Rehabilitation, 12,* 40–53.

Citation	Purpose	Level/Design/Participants	Intervention/Outcome Measures	Results	Comments	Conclusions
Van Ort & Phillips, 1995	The purpose of this study was to evaluate the efficacy of two nursing interventions, one contextual and one behavioral, designed to promote functional feeding and to maintain adequate nutritional status of a sample of older adults with dementia living in a long-term-care setting.	**Level III** 1-group, repeated measures **Participants** 8 participants from a secure nursing unit of a large residential geriatric center. Participants met the following criteria: (a) Required feeding assistance by a caregiver (b) Were able to sit in a chair for feeding (c) Were responsive to human interaction (d) Were not usually restrained during feeding (e) Were not usually combative One participant was dropped from the study after baseline data were taken because the participant did not met the first criteria. Participants ranged in age from 65 to 93.	**Intervention** Contextual intervention was provided for all participants for 2 wk. The intervention involved creating a context for feeding that encouraged self-feeding and a positive atmosphere. 4 participants were randomly selected to receive the Behavioral Intervention, which involved cues to encourage and reinforce feeding. **Outcome Measures** *Baseline:* ■ Weight measured in pounds using a spring scale in the morning before to breakfast ■ MMSE *Time 1:* Two complete lunches and two dinners were videotaped for all participants and all participants were weighed. *Time 2:* Videotaping and weights were used at the end of 2 weeks of contextual intervention. *Time 3:* Weights obtained at the end of behavioral intervention. *Time 4:* Baseline measures repeated 1 month after intervention.	All results were presented anecdotally, with no supporting data, although the authors stated that repeated measures ANOVA were used to test the hypotheses. Both the contextual and behavioral interventions resulted in feeding-related interpersonal contact between residents and feeders. Both interventions resulted in a better match between the functional abilities of the participant and the level of assistance offered by the feeder. Participants' weights were maintained through all phases of the study.	Results were reported descriptively (in narrative form), making it difficult to know the degree to which the interventions had any influence on the outcomes. The sample size was small with no power calculation. An unequal number of participants received the contextual ($n = 3$) versus behavioral ($n = 4$) intervention. Only 1 videotape (randomly selected) for each participant was transcribed and coded. Data from transcriptions were not reported.	The authors concluded that both the contextual and behavioral interventions can promote self-feeding, and no decrease in participants' weight occurred. However, it is difficult to conclude the relative value of these interventions without supporting data.

Van Ort, S., & Phillips, L. R. (1995). Nursing intervention to promote functional feeding. *Journal of Gerontological Nursing, 21*, 6–14.

(continued)

EVIDENCE TABLE: What is the evidence for the effect of interventions designed to establish, modify, and maintain activities of daily living (ADLs), instrumental activities of daily living (IADLs), leisure, and social participation on the quality of life, health and wellness, and client and caregiver satisfaction for persons with dementia? *(continued)*

Author/Year	Study Objectives	Level/Design/ Participants	Intervention and Outcome Measures	Results	Study Limitations	Implications for Occupational Therapy
Yang, Mann, Nochajski, & Tomita, 1997	This is a follow-up study to gain a better understanding of the need for and use of assistive devices by participants with cognitive impairment. This study provides a follow-up on the use of current assistive devices by participants in the Nochajski et al. (1996) study and including caregivers' perspectives on previous occupational therapy interventions.	Level III 1-group pre–post study *n* = 10 could be followed up from original study of *n* = 20. 5 were living at home; 2 had moved to a nursing home; and 3 had died. Informal caregivers provided the information for the 3 participants that were deceased. Of the 7 participants still alive at the time of follow-up—Age ranged from 72–92; 85.7% White 66.7% completed high school 50% reported incomes <$10,000 100% married	Intervention Follow-up visits were conducted 1–2 years after the occupational therapy intervention. Interviews took place in the participants' residence, and the investigators readministered previously used assessments. Outcome Measures ■ OARS health status questions ■ FIM ■ OARS IADLs ■ MMSE ■ Zarit Caregiver Burden Scale ■ Use of assistive devices	There were declines in FIM, IADL, and MMSE scores from initial study to follow-up. At time of follow-up, the mean total owned devices dropped from 10 after occupational therapy intervention to 8.6 devices (*n* = 5 participants still living at home). The mean total used declined from 8.5 to 6.3. Standard deviations were large. At follow-up, 58% of the total devices were used. Mean satisfaction ratings were down to 6.0 at follow-up (compared with 7.8 at time of intervention). 6 of 8 caregivers reported that the occupational therapy interventions were helpful (numeric ratings not provided).	The study was only able to follow up with half of the original study, and of the 10, only 7 were alive. Therefore, only descriptive data could be reported, making it difficult to draw conclusions from this study. The authors stated that due to the significant decline in health, mental, and functional status from the initial study to this follow-up study, participant recruitment was challenging and resulted in a sample size Caregiver data were not reported numerically.	Given the exploratory nature of this study and the small sample size, future research is needed to further explore the usefulness of occupational therapy interventions for persons with cognitive impairment and the perceived satisfaction with the assistive devices provided as intervention. The authors highlighted that there is an opportunity for occupational therapists to provide training for home health care aids; however, future research exploring the potential benefits is required.

Yang, J., Mann, W. C., Nochajski, S., & Tomita, M. R. (1997). Use of assistive devices among elders with cognitive impairment: A follow-up study. *Topics in Geriatric Rehabilitation, 13,* 13–31.

Instrumental activities of daily living (IADLs)

		Intervention		
Avila, Bottino, Carvalho, Santos, Seral, & Miotto, 2004	A pilot study was undertaken to ■ Explore the effects of neuropsychological rehabilitation on people with mild AD, and ■ Report on tests and scales used to evaluate and re-evaluate cognitive status, efficiency of implicit and explicit memory techniques and IADL training of patients with AD in neuropsychological rehabilitation programs.	**Level III** Before and after **Participants** 1 man and 4 women diagnosed with probable AD, mildly impaired. Caregivers were also involved. All participants also on Rivastigmine, 6–12 mg, for ≥3 mo.	14 week period, including 60-min. weekly group sessions and 30-min. weekly individual sessions. Errorless learning technique was used throughout. Program consisted of memory training—motor movement, verbal associations, and categorization and IADL training: telephone use, diary use, and food prep. **Outcome Measures** ■ MMSE ■ Montgomery-Alsberg depression rating scale ■ Hamilton anxiety scale ■ Interview to determine deterioration in daily function, functional test (unpublished, Avila), memory of daily living questionnaire ■ Quality of life questionnaire ■ Neuropsychological test battery	Continuous scores of cognitive tests and scales before and after test were compared using the Wilcoxan test. Modest improvement was noted on most scales after treatment (including quality of life). No improvement was noted on the memory of daily living questionnaire patient. Quality of life improved for patients and caregivers, but the changes were not statistically significant ($p = .60$, $p = .83$, respectively). The only statistically significant improvement was noted in the functional test.	The only scale showing a statistically significant outcome has not been published. Sample size is quite small ($n = 5$), suggesting limited power to detect statistically significant differences. No control group. Difficult to disentangle the benefits of rivastigmine vs. neuropsychological rehabilitation vs. caregiver orientation vs. Hawthorne effect.	Neuropsychological rehabilitation may have a place in treating mildly impaired people with probable Alzheimer disease. This study does not show definitive results, but a trend toward improvement in cognition, ADL function, and psychiatric symptoms after an neuropsychological rehabilitation program. It must be noted that this strategy is combined with pharmacological intervention. The study points out the advantage of using implicit memory strategies in people with AD, because implicit memory is still intact early in the disease. It also suggests specific treatment for specific problems to reduce the need to generalize strategies.

Avila, R., Bottino, C. M., Carvalho, I. A., Santos, C. B., Seral, C., & Miotto, E. C. (2004). Neuropsychological rehabilitation of memory deficits and activities of daily living in patients with Alzheimer's disease: A pilot study. *Brazilian Journal of Medical and Biological Research, 37,* 1721–1729.

(continued)

EVIDENCE TABLE: What is the evidence for the effect of interventions designed to establish, modify, and maintain activities of daily living (ADLs), instrumental activities of daily living (IADLs), leisure, and social participation on the quality of life, health and wellness, and client and caregiver satisfaction for persons with dementia? *(continued)*

Author/Year	Study Objectives	Level/Design/ Participants	Intervention and Outcome Measures	Results	Study Limitations	Implications for Occupational Therapy
Dooley & Hinojosa, 2004	The overarching objective of the research was to determine the extent to which adherence to occupational therapy recommendations increases the quality of life of people with dementia as well as decrease the level of burden experienced by their family caregivers.	Level I Pretest–posttest control group design with random assignment to groups. Participants 40 participants with AD who attended an outpatient memory disorders clinic. Men = 16 (40%) Women = 24 (60%)	Intervention • Home occupational therapy assessment and recommendations using the AIF, the AAL-AD Burden Interview, and PSMS to develop recommendations • Telephone follow-up conducted at 1 mo (although the average was 2.3 mo) Both groups received the initial visit and assessment. The intervention group received written recommendations and a second home visit to review the written report and discuss implementations of recommendations. The control group participants received the written recommendations in the mail after the telephone follow-up. Outcome Measures ■ Zarit Burden Inventory ■ AAL-AD (described as a quality of life measure) ■ PSMS	Using multiple ANCOVA, significant group effects were found for caregiver burden, positive affect, activity frequency, and self-care status ($p < .001$). Bivariate analyses identified the contribution of each dependent variable to the overall effect, with caregiver burden ($p < .001$), positive affect ($p = .015$), and self-care status ($p = .03$) statistically significant, but activity frequency was not statistically significant ($p = .58$).	Follow-up procedures were frequently delayed from the original 1 mo planned in the procedure. This may have resulted in differences in recall. Telephone follow-up was not always done by a blind assessor, which may have resulted in bias. Study design is confusing in the description; it is not clear why the authors have not described this as a randomized trial. The intervention/ recommendations are not described in enough detail to replicate the study. The authors describe the AAL–AD as a quality-of-life scale, but its focus is on engagement in and enjoyment of activities.	The results of this study suggest that occupational therapy recommendations based on in-home assessment with clients with dementia and their caregivers followed by a home visit may improve quality of life and decrease caregiver burden. While promising, further information is needed to understand the intervention in more detail and to demonstrate the need for the home visit to improve the implementation of recommendations.

Dooley, N. R., & Hinojosa, J. (2004). Improving quality of life for persons with Alzheimer's disease and their family caregivers: Brief occupational therapy intervention. *American Journal of Occupational Therapy, 58,* 561–569.

| Fitzsimmons & Buettner, 2003 | The objective was to examine the effect of a therapeutic cooking program on agitated behaviors, passive behaviors, and physiological processes when provided to older adults with dementia. | Level I
Pretest–posttest experimental design (delayed intervention control group)

This was a substudy of a larger trial focusing on therapeutic recreation interventions.

Participants
12 participants (all women) with a diagnosis of dementia who resided within an assisted living center on a locked SCU in Florida. | Intervention
Therapeutic cooking group were offered 5 days/wk for 2 wk for approximately 1 hour. Control group participants were involved in normal facility activities, followed by another 2 wks in the therapeutic recreational cooking group.

Outcome Measures
■ Cohen Mansfield Agitation Inventory, Passivity in Dementia Scale
■ Biograph system (blood pressure variability and heart rate) | There was a significant (improvement) reduction in agitation in the intervention group ($p < .000$) compared with the control (NS change). Passivity decreased significantly in the intervention group ($p < .001$) compared to the control group ($p = .586$).

Blood pressure (as a proxy for health) increased as engagement increased, and decreased as agitation decreased ($p < .067$). | Small sample size is not justified; only women were included.

Limited time to offer the intervention (2 wk).

Analyses are not well described.

The notion of engaging people with dementia in functional activities such as cooking has face validity. It appears that the intervention had statistically significant effects on behavioral outcomes, but not for the health outcomes (blood pressure and heart rate). Although this may not be surprising, it is difficult to make conclusions about the outcomes of this study in light of the focused question. |

Fitzsimmons, S., & Buettner, L. L. (2003). A therapeutic cooking program for older adults with dementia: Effects on agitation and apathy. *American Journal of Recreation Therapy, 2,* 23–33.

(continued)

EVIDENCE TABLE: What is the evidence for the effect of interventions designed to establish, modify, and maintain activities of daily living (ADLs), instrumental activities of daily living (IADLs), leisure, and social participation on the quality of life, health and wellness, and client and caregiver satisfaction for persons with dementia? (continued)

Author/Year	Study Objectives	Level/Design/ Participants	Intervention and Outcome Measures	Results	Study Limitations	Implications for Occupational Therapy
Graff, Vernooij-Dassen, Hoefnagels, Dekker, & de Witte, 2003	The aim of the pilot study was to explore the effects of an occupational therapy intervention on the performance of daily activities by older individuals with mild to moderate cognitive impairments and on the sense of competence of their primary caregivers.	<u>Level III</u> Single group pretest–posttest <u>Participants</u> $n = 12$ older adults with mild to moderate cognitive impairment and their caregivers. Average age of participants = 79.9 years and average age of caregivers = 56.6 years. Participants were discharged from the Department of Geriatrics of a medical center in the Netherlands.	<u>Intervention</u> Client-centered occupational therapy (2 wk intervention at the hospital and 5 wk at home); 2×/ week (maximum of 10 occupational therapy home visits) <u>Outcome Measures</u> ■ AMPS ■ IDDD ■ Sense of Competence Questionnaire ■ BCRS ■ COPM	Between baseline (before any occupational therapy intervention (T0)) and after 7 wk of occupational therapy intervention (T1), almost all of the outcome measures for older individuals with cognitive impairment improved significantly: AMPS motor ($p = 0.014$), AMPS process ($p = .005$), IDDD performance ($p = .032$), IDDD initiative ($p = .165$), COPM performance ($p = .009$), COPM satisfaction ($p = .002$), BCRS scores ($p = .394$), and the sense of competence among primary caregivers showed a significant improvement ($p = .022$).	Small sample with no control group to compare to effect of interventions is a limitation. It is difficult to know which strategies were most frequently applied and how much environmental intervention was used compared with involving the person with dementia in IADL or other activities.	The results of this pilot study indicated that older clients' motor and process skills and self-perception in occupational performance improved and that they needed less help. In terms of the focused question, satisfaction with performance improved significantly. The sense of competence of their primary caregivers also improved. This study provides preliminary evidence for the effectiveness of occupational therapy in older individuals with cognitive impairments and their primary caregivers, which should be tested in a randomized controlled trial.

Graff, M. J. L., Vernooij-Dassen, M. J. F., Hoefnagels, W. H. L., Dekker, J., & de Witte, L. P. (2003). Occupational therapy at home for older individuals with mild to moderate cognitive impairments and their primary caregivers: A pilot study. *OTJR: Occupation, Participation and Health, 23*, 155–164.

Graff, Vernooij-Dassen, Thijssen, Dekker, Hoefnagels, & Rikkert, 2006	The objective was to evaluate the effectiveness of a community occupational therapy intervention. Primary outcomes of the study (patient function and caregiver sense of competence) were the focus of a different publication. This article focused on secondary outcomes, including client and caregiver health status, mood, quality of life, and sense of control.	Level I RCT Participants 135 people with mild to moderate dementia and their caregivers, recruited through an outpatient memory clinic or geriatric day program.	Intervention Client-centered occupational therapy was offered in 10 1-hr sessions over 5 weeks. 4 sessions focused on identifying occupational performance issues and goal setting; 6 focused on supporting clients and caregivers to implement compensation and environmental strategies. Outcome Measures ■ Dementia Quality of Life Scale ■ GHQ-12	Clients with dementia: At 6 wk, there were statistically significant differences in favor of the intervention group for the overall and all subscales of the Dementia Quality of Life Scale ($p < .0001$). At 12 wk, all differences continued to be statistically significant, although some p values went up, suggesting the differences between groups were not as great at 12 wk. Statistically significant differences were in favor of the intervention group for health status at 6 and 12 weeks ($p < .0001$). Caregivers: At 6 wk, there were statistically significant differences in favor of the intervention group for overall quality-of-life scores ($p < .0001$) and all but one subscale (negative affect). At 12 wk, results were similar but 2 Dementia Quality-of-Life Scale subscales (positive and negative affect) were not significant. There was a statistically significant difference in favor of the intervention for health status of caregivers at 6 and 12 wk ($p < .0001$).	Control group did not receive an attention placebo, so there is some chance that the differences were related to increased attention. Although blind assessments were conducted, 18%–20% of assessors were unblinded. Because few studies report the rate at which unblinding occurs, it is difficult to know if this resulted in bias. Participants recruited from a medical center; may have been different than the typical population of people with mild to moderate dementia.	The results of this study are very positive in demonstrating the effectiveness of a community-based occupational therapy intervention for people with mild and moderate dementia. Details about the intervention are available in another publication by Graff et al., 2006. The intervention is based on client-centered principles and used a number of well-accepted approaches to gain information about occupational performance issues. The amount of training provided to the study therapists may limit applicability. It is not clear whether that degree of training is required for broad implementation. Further, remuneration for the intervention may be challenging to access in some countries. Cost effectiveness could be assessed in future research.

(continued)

Graff, M. J. L., Vernooij-Dassen, M. J. M., Thijssen, M., Dekker, J., Hoefnagels, W. H. L., & Rikkert, M. G. M. (2007). Effects of community occupational therapy on quality of life, mood, and health status in dementia patients and their caregivers: A randomized controlled trial. *Journals of Gerontology (Medical Sciences), 62A*, 1002–1009.

EVIDENCE TABLE: What is the evidence for the effect of interventions designed to establish, modify, and maintain activities of daily living (ADLs), instrumental activities of daily living (IADLs), leisure, and social participation on the quality of life, health and wellness, and client and caregiver satisfaction for persons with dementia? *(continued)*

Author/Year	Study Objectives	Level/Design/ Participants	Intervention and Outcome Measures	Results	Study Limitations	Implications for Occupational Therapy
Topo, Jylha, & Laine, 2002	The purpose of the study was to understand the role of the telephone in everyday communications of people with dementia and their caregivers, and to evaluate the usefulness of an easy-to-use telephone for this group.	<u>Level IV</u> Descriptive case studies <u>Participants</u> 6 community-dwelling residents with mild to moderate dementia. Participants exhibited current difficulty operating the telephone. Participants were recommended for the study by a dementia care coordinator, social worker, or head of a dementia day care centre.	<u>Intervention</u> Implementation of a telephone with photographs and programmed numbers. Test period lasted 2 mo. <u>Outcome Measures</u> ■ Study designed questionnaire: Families were asked to complete the questionnaire 10× over 2 mo. Questions focused on the use of the phone. ■ CDR ■ Telephone section of the IADLs scale ■ Interview at end of study	After phone introduction: *Participant A:* Abilities remained the same *Participant B:* Able to dial a few well-known numbers *Participant C:* Abilities remained the same *Participant D:* Able to dial a few well-known numbers *Participant E:* Able to dial a few well-known numbers *Participant F:* Able to answer the telephone but not dial Families reported increased satisfaction with the telephones through interviews.	Participants with dementia were interviewed in front of family members, which may have complicated results. The study had a small sample size with detailed description. It is unclear how interview data were analyzed or if data presented are representative of the whole sample. There is a limited ability to generalize findings from a small sample with descriptive findings.	Few conclusions can be drawn from this study. Programmable phones are an assistive device that occupational therapists can consider when working with people with dementia and their families. However, this study has not demonstrated their effectiveness. Rather it suggests that it may improve telephone use abilities, and satisfaction. Further evaluation of such devices is needed.

Topo, P., Jylha, M., & Laine, J. (2002). Can the telephone-using abilities of people with dementia be promoted? An evaluation of a simple-to-use telephone. *Technology and Disability, 14,* 3–13.

| Buettner, 1999 | The objective was to determine if age-and-stage appropriate sensorimotor recreational items

■ Positively affect frequency and quality of visits?

■ Increase the time spent by residents in purposeful activities and decrease agitated behavior?

■ Can be identified for residents at each stage of the disease? | Level III
Clinical cross-over

Phase I: (pilot test)
3 mo testing of sensorimotor items in a unrelated facility
Phase II: (Study)
2 different 40-bed DSCUs were used. Residents in 1 received intervention for 6 mo on then 6 mo off. Residents in the other facility received the same intervention in the opposite order.

Participants
55 residents with a dementia diagnosis (81% women; average age 87.4 years). 43 staff participated in a survey component. 51 family interviews (20 from 1 nursing home and 31 from the other). | Intervention
Pilot: 30 handmade sensorimotor recreational items were designed and tested for residents of different functioning levels.
Phase II: Intervention items with instruction sheets were given to family members and community volunteers. Residents could freely choose items from an open cart. Volunteers were provided with a 30-min Dementia Education Program. Staff were provided with a weekly 10-min in-service at shift change to introduce new items.

Outcome Measures
■ The Family Interview Form to determine perceived quality of family visits and use of recreational items
■ An informal count of community volunteer involvement
■ Residents and staff assessed at baseline, 2 midpoints, and end-point of study
■ Families interviewed at midpoint and end-point | 23 items were found to be therapeutically valuable and acceptable for nursing home use in Phase I.

Frequency of family visits (Site 1: $p < .006$, Site 2: $p < .000$), use of: recreational items (Site 1: $p < .001$, Site 2: $p < .000$), and satisfaction with visits (Site 1: $p < .011$, Site 2: $p < .000$) were higher during the intervention period. | Study lacks specific details about the timing, frequency, duration, and who delivered the intervention.

Statistical analysis is sketchy and confusing. | Although the use of sensorimotor recreational items is primarily a therapeutic recreational activity, occupational therapists are also concerned with social participation in leisure activities. As part of the team, occupational therapists are skilled in assessing residents' level of functioning and determining the type of sensorimotor activity that is appropriate for the staff or family to use during their interaction with the resident. The evidence from this study suggests that by providing an opportunity for family to engage in meaningful activity with their family member, quality, satisfaction, and number of visits may increase. The study also infers that the intervention can be used throughout the progression of the disease process, with certain items being more appropriate than others depending on the stage of illness. |

Buettner, L. L. (1999). Simple pleasures: A multilevel sensorimotor intervention for nursing home residents with dementia. *American Journal of Alzheimer's Disease, 14,* 41–52

(continued)

EVIDENCE TABLE: What is the evidence for the effect of interventions designed to establish, modify, and maintain activities of daily living (ADLs), instrumental activities of daily living (IADLs), leisure, and social participation on the quality of life, health and wellness, and client and caregiver satisfaction for persons with dementia? *(continued)*

Author/Year	Study Objectives	Level/Design/ Participants	Intervention and Outcome Measures	Results	Study Limitations	Implications for Occupational Therapy
Chung, 2004	The objective was to explore the states of well-being of long-term care residents with dementia when participating in their usual activity pattern. Subquestions: ■ What types of activity did individuals engage in? ■ Were the patterns of activity engagement different across different stages of dementia? ■ What were the states of well-being for individuals at different stages of dementia? ■ How did the states of well-being relate to the time spent in different types of activities?	Level III Cross-sectional _Participants_ 43 residents with a medical diagnosis of dementia or a dementia-related disorder, living for > 6 mo in 1 of 2 nursing homes in Hong Kong. Average age 81 (67% women) Participants classified by a medical practitioner according to their cognitive and functional impairment using the CDR: CDR1 = mild impairment (*n* = 22); CDR2 = moderate (*n* = 15), CDR3 = severe (*n* = 6)	_Intervention_ Occupational therapy, social work, and nursing involved in planning of activities but not clearly outlined. One measure was used to classify observations: Dementia Care Mapping. Observation of activity patterns in natural environments. Activity classification divided into two types: Type I indicates activities with a potential for interaction. Type II is the opposite. Mapping sessions were done weekly with 4–5 participants observed for a period of not < 6 hours; all sessions completed within 3 months. Two scores were generated: ■ A code representing the type of activity participants engage in ■ A well-being/ill-being value	ANOVA showed statistically significant differences of time spent in different activities among the 3 CDR groups: therapeutic/leisure (*p* < .001); ADLs (*p* < .001); mobility and interaction (*p* = .01); passive (*p* < .001) and negative (*p* = .001). 2-way ANOVA showed no interaction effect of the sites or the cognitive impairment on the 5 types of activities. Kruskal-Wallis test indicated significant difference in the well-being values among the 3 CDR groups ($\chi^2 = 27.01$, *p* < .001). Significant positive correlations were shown to exist between well-being and Type I activities (*p* < .001). Significant negative correlations were found between the state of well-being and time spent in Type II activities (*p* < .001).	Convenience sample was used; therefore, generalization is limited. The sample size was small, especially because the total sample was further divided into groups. There was a lack of accounting for confounding factors in the social or physical environment. This is a descriptive study only, and therefore interpretation of results must be cautious.	"The most important concern of patients is to participate as actively as possible for as long as possible" (p. 29). Study helps to clarify patterns in activity at different levels of cognitive impairment. May assist in planning and structuring appropriate activities for clients at that level. This study will assist occupational therapists to tailor individual activity profiles and look for methods to transition skills from 1 level of performance to another, to support and maintain engagement and sense of well-being. Occupational therapists may also be able to use information to educate and facilitate caregivers on how to maintain participation. Program development goals and need for funding for staffing to carry out programming specific to individual needs can be supported if the evidence from this study is supported by future higher level research.

Chung, J. C. C. (2004). Activity participation and well-being of people with dementia in long-term-care settings. *OTJR: Occupation, Participation and Health, 24,* 22–31.

| Clair & Ebberts, 1997 | The objective was to determine whether music therapy has an effect on the relationship between caregivers and care receivers in the following:

• Caregivers' perception of feelings of
(a) depression,
(b) burden,
(c) positive and negative affect,
(d) self-reported health, and
(e) satisfaction with visits

• Frequency of engagement as indicated by initiated physical contact, or touch, and response to physical contact, or touch

• Frequency of participation in meaningful activities, including
(a) conversation,
(b) singing,
(c) drumming, and
(d) dancing. | Level III
Pretest–posttest

Participants

15 significant others, who regularly visited persons diagnosed with severe dementia, agreed to participate in the study at residential care homes. 12 completed the study. Participants were assigned to groups of 2 to 4 couples. | Intervention

8 music therapy sessions 2× weekly for 4 wk at the residential care homes. Sessions occurred at the same time and day of week. Each session was structured by a music therapist and consisted of 10 min each of initial conversation; singing; ballroom, folk, or chair dancing; rhythm participation using drums; and follow-up conversation with consideration given to individual music preferences, physical abilities, culture, and the like.

Outcomes Measures

• Boundary Ambiguity Scale for Caregivers of Patients with Dementia
• Montgomery and Borgatta Burden Scale
• The Hamilton Rating Scale for Depression
• The Positive and Negative Affect Scale
• Self-reported health
• Visit Satisfaction Survey completed before first session and after final session | Results were analyzed using 2-tailed t tests and found not to be significant for any measure except satisfaction with visits ($p = .017$). Caregivers' measures of depression, burden, positive and negative affect, and self-reported health did not change. Caregivers' engagement in participation was significantly higher in singing and rhythm playing compared with conversation. Care receivers had statistically significant difference in participation during rhythm playing vs. conversation. Caregivers initiated touch more frequently than their care receivers, but care receivers were more responsive to touch than their caregivers. | Sample size was small.

There was a referral bias because the caregivers who were selected to attend were already highly involved with the care receiver.

This was a convenience sample with no randomization nor control group comparison.

No demographic data were provided about the caregivers or care receivers.

Outcome measures were not well known and there was no reporting of psychometric properties. | Music participation provides sensory stimulation and meaningful engagement and is an intervention that can be implemented and tailored specifically to an individual's abilities. Although this intervention was carried out by a music therapist, occupational therapists also have the skills necessary to identify the specific benefits that might be derived for an individual and provide this intervention to restore and maintain purposeful interaction between caregivers and care receivers. They can also advocate the inclusion of music into leisure programming. |

Clair, A. A., & Ebberts, A. (1997). The effects of music therapy on interactions between family caregivers and their care receivers with late stage dementia. *Journal of Music Therapy, 34,* 148–164.

(continued)

Author/Year	Study Objectives	Level/Design/ Participants	Intervention and Outcome Measures	Results	Study Limitations	Implications for Occupational Therapy
Colling & Buettner, 2002	The objective was to ascertain whether age-and-stage appropriate sensorimotor recreational items, constructed by families and volunteers: ■ Positively affect frequency and quality of visits ■ Increase time spent in purposeful activity and decrease disturbing behavior ■ Are most appropriate at different functional levels and behavioral needs.	<u>Level III</u> Clinical cross-over design conducted at 2 nursing homes on 40-bed SCUs for 6 mo with a 1-mo "wash-out" period between sites. <u>Participants</u> The sample size is not reported; the sample is not described.	<u>Intervention</u> 30 fabricated recreational items were used during visits with residents at a nursing home <u>Outcome Measures</u> Data collected through random videotaping, family interviews, direct observation, and questionnaires using the: ■ CMAI—completed at 4 time points ■ MMSE ■ GDS ■ MDS medication listing ■ Number of visits— using a unit log-in system ■ Volunteer count	The Simple Pleasures Project increased the number of volunteers and increased visiting of families and friends ($p < .006$, $p < .000$ at the 2 sites, respectively) and the satisfaction with visits was significantly improved ($p < .001$, $p < .000$). Families at both sites reported using items significantly more ($p < .000$, $p < .001$). Agitation was significantly reduced ($p < .001$) during the intervention period at Site 1 but only slightly reduced at Site 2 (p value not reported).	The sample included in the study is not defined or described, making it difficult to consider generalizability. Contextual issues, including environmental and client characteristics affect the outcome directly, and they may moderate the intervention effects. These factors are not reported in any way. There is no clear report of interventions and no reporting of data collected. Statistical analyses are not described.	Although this study indicates that certain Simple Pleasure items were found to decrease disturbing behaviors and increase frequency and satisfaction of visitors, it is difficult to draw conclusions. The concepts underlying the Simple Pleasures program have face validity, and the article describes its theoretical underpinnings. Further evidence would be needed to endorse this intervention. If adopted and evaluated, occupational therapists may play a role in determining which items are appropriate for the resident as well as educating families and volunteers in the use of these items.

Colling, K. B., & Buettner, L. L. (2002). Simple pleasures: Interventions from the need-driven dementia-compromised behavior model. *Journal of Gerontological Nursing, 28,* 16–20.

Crispi & Heitner, 2002	The objective was to present families with a series of kits that they could use in their visits, to have family members evaluate the kits, and to replicate the program independently to demonstrate that it could be useful in other settings and facilities.	Level IV Descriptive study using feedback from family participants. Participants 29 families were asked to use the activity kits, over a 12-wk period, in visits with their family member with dementia. Participants were family members of nursing home residents with dementia. Participants were excluded if they had a significant psychiatric history, unstable medical illness, or cognitive abilities	Intervention 10 kits were developed on the basis of different stages of ability. 4 were eliminated during pilot period. Outcome Measure Outcome measure was an evaluation form that ranked, on a scale of 1–5: resident involvement, kit's contribution to the visit, over all value of kit, value of each item.	Puzzles and reminiscence kits contributed most to the quality of the visits. Sounds of the past and card games contributed the least. Active music and puzzles were rated most valuable. Card games were the least valuable. Families reported that the kits improved the quality of visits and improved quality of life of the residents.	Weak study design	Although the activity kit intervention may be seen more as recreational, occupational therapists can have input on development of kits at various levels of cognitive difficulty. This can provide options for visits and help improve the quality of the interaction for both family and caregivers.

Crispi, E. L., & Heitner, G. (2002). An activity-based intervention for caregivers and residents with dementia in nursing homes. *Activities, Adaptation, and Aging, 26*, 61–72.

(continued)

Author/Year	Study Objectives	Level/Design/Participants	Intervention and Outcome Measures	Results	Study Limitations	Implications for Occupational Therapy
Gitlin, Winter, Burke, Chernett, Dennis, & Hauck, 2008	The objective was to evaluate the effectiveness of the TAP, which was designed to ■ Reduce behavior disturbances in people with dementia ■ Enhance patient engagement ■ Reduce caregiver burden ■ Improve caregiver mastery, self-efficacy, and use of communication and simplification strategies. The study also examined differences in outcomes for caregivers experiencing depression compared with those not experiencing depression.	Level Randomized controlled pilot study Participants 60 community-dwelling people with dementia and their resident caregivers Participants with dementia: Mean age = 79.4; 56.7% male; 76.1% White; mean MMSE score = 11.6 Caregivers: Mean age = 65.4; 11.7% male; 76.1% White; 61.7% spouse caregivers	Intervention Tailored Activities Program (TAP): On the basis of the initial assessment and interview, 3 activities were identified for each participant and a written activity prescription was developed to match the individual's capabilities and decrease environmental demands. (Note: Most of the activities fit under the leisure area of occupation, although others were IADLs, ADLs, social participation.) Intervention was 4 mo with 6 visits to the client/caregiver home and 2 telephone contacts. Control: Wait listed for 4 mo—no attention control Outcomes Measures ■ Quality of Life–AD ■ Acceptability of TAP (data on other behavioral and caregiver measures were also collected)	Quality of Life: There were no significant differences between people with dementia in the intervention and control group (p = .095) after 4 mo. Acceptability of TAP ■ 69.6% of the patients were reported as being engaged "very much." ■ Only 6.5% refused participation. ■ 84.8% of the caregivers indicated that the intervention was very useful. ■ 89.1% of the caregivers indicated that the intervention had a positive effect. ■ 100% of the caregivers demonstrated understanding of strategies somewhat or very much. ■ Only 2.2% did not use recommended activities.	There may have been attention bias: control group participants received no intervention. All were volunteers were based on advertisements. The sample size may not have had adequate power to detect difference in quality of life (but note that behavioral disturbances were the primary outcomes). Co-intervention was not addressed (in particular use of medications). The number and training of interventionists was not described. Acceptability of TAP was based on 1 rating by interventionist and caregiver at the end of the 4-mo intervention.	An intervention that tailors activities to the individual strengths and interests of people with dementia is accepted by people with dementia and their caregivers; caregivers also reported that the intervention had a positive effect. Quality-of-life outcomes were not demonstrated to be positively affected in the intervention group compared to the control group after 4 mo, but other behavioral and caregiver outcomes suggested positive preliminary findings. The intervention is grounded in client-centered occupational therapy practice, with emphasis on activity analysis and modification.

Gitlin, L. N., Winter, L., Burke, J., Chernett, N., Dennis, M. P., & Hauck, W. W. (2008). Tailored activities to manage neuropsychiatric behaviors in persons with dementia and reduce caregiver burden: A randomized pilot study. American Journal of Geriatric Psychiatry, 16, 229–239.

Pool, 2001	Level IV	Intervention	Allen Cognitive Level:	Study lacks a control	This is a low-level study

Study	Design	Intervention / Outcome Measures	Results	Limitations	Comments
Pool, 2001	The objective was to describe the development of a person-centered model of care based on the implementation of meaningful activity.	<u>Intervention</u> Activity therapist spent 30 min 3×/wk for 4 wk with participants choosing an activity from 5 standardized structured activities. 1-on-1 time and attention control: Activity therapist spent 30 min, 3×/wk for 4 wk with participants, either conversing or participating in unstructured, relaxed activities. <u>Outcome Measures</u> ■ Neuropsychiatric Inventory NPI apathy domain and total NPI score ■ Alzheimer's Disease Related Quality of Life scale ■ Copper Ridge Activity Index	<i>Allen Cognitive Level:</i> 3 of 7 participants showed improvement (not described) Cognitive Response Affective Index: There was a modest decrease in the need for cueing in the control ("one-to-one") group ($p = .027$)	Study lacks a control group with no intervention. There was rater bias, because raters knew participants were receiving some intervention. Limited information is available on reliability, validity, and responsiveness to change of outcome measures. The participants were not clearly reported in terms of ethnicity or gender.	This is a low-level study that is really more of a narrative report about a change in philosophy that coincided with the introduction of an activity program. More rigorous reporting of the outcome measure and more rigorous evaluation of the intervention would be useful for occupational therapy because the method involves use of an occupational performance profile to assist with planning individualized activity programs. As the study is presented, it is not possible to draw any conclusions related to this program. Although it makes clinical sense to be able to evaluate remaining activity performance to optimize participation in self-care and leisure, more rigorous study and reporting are necessary.
	<u>Level IV</u> Pretest–posttest design <u>Participants</u> 37 residents of a care facility with dementia according to DSM-IV. No report of demographic data, drop-outs, selection criteria of participants.				

Pool, J. (2001). Making contact: An activity-based model of care. *Journal of Dementia Care, 9*, 24–26.

(continued)

EVIDENCE TABLE: What is the evidence for the effect of interventions designed to establish, modify, and maintain activities of daily living (ADLs), instrumental activities of daily living (IADLs), leisure, and social participation on the quality of life, health and wellness, and client and caregiver satisfaction for persons with dementia? (continued)

Author/Year	Study Objectives	Level/Design/ Participants	Intervention and Outcome Measures	Results	Study Limitations	Implications for Occupational Therapy
Rentz, 2002	The objective was to describe and present the results of a pilot project: an outcomes-based evaluation of an art program (Memories in the Making) for individuals with dementing illness.	<u>Level IV</u> Descriptive study <u>Participants</u> *n* = 41 Participants were chosen from 4 adult day programs, 1 assisted-living facility, and 1 dementia-specific nursing home. 41 artist participants and 6 staff observers were chosen. No indication was given for reasons for selection of participants. No descriptors were provided for participants.	<u>Intervention</u> An art program for individuals with dementia (early and middle stages) was the intervention. The intervention was guided by skilled artist facilitators. Participants used watercolors and acrylics to express themselves. The process allowed them to recreate a memory, tell a story, and enjoy being involved in creating something of value. <u>Outcome Measures</u> Affect state and self-esteem: Tool was developed by staff that operationally defined both domains in terms of specific, observable indicators. Indicators were rated on a 4 point-Likert scale.	Indicators suggested that individuals always or some of the time worked with sustained attention, had a pleasurable sensory experience, experienced pleasure (as evidenced by laughter and relaxed body posture), and verbalized feeling good about themselves and their accomplishments. The authors felt that 1 of the most positive indicators of well-being (engagement) confirmed that 83% of participants had sustained attention for 30–45 min. They felt spontaneous comments of participants offered good insights.	The authors clearly state that this was a pilot project to determine appropriate evaluation for a program and was not designed as a research study. As such, the results can only be used to describe this particular situation. Demographic data were not provided. The operational definition of the indicators in the measurement tool is unclear. No assessment of interrater reliability when 6 raters are contributing was provided.	There are limited implications for occupational therapy, in large part because this is a very preliminary exploration of a specialized program. This type of program is typically conducted by therapeutic recreation or art therapy. However, the occupational therapist may be involved with the occupation of recreation and may assess the client's appropriateness for the group or help establish the client's strengths and remaining abilities to facilitate success within the program. It would be useful to have a valid and reliable tool to measure well-being in clients with dementia where self-report can often be difficult.

Rentz, C. A. (2002). Memories in the making: Outcome-based evaluation of an art program for individuals with dementing illnesses. *American Journal of Alzheimer's Disease and Other Dementias, 17*, 175–181.

Social Participation

Bourgeois & Mason, 1996	The objective was to evaluate the effects of memory wallet use on the conversational behaviors of people with dementia working with volunteers in an adult day care setting, to examine the effect of the memory wallet intervention on volunteers' conversational behaviors, and to consider feasibility of assigning responsibility for a client activity to volunteers.	<u>Level IV</u> Single-case design; multiple baselines with replication across participants <u>Participants</u> *Day care clients:* 4 clients with dementia attending an adult day care setting. *Volunteers:* Three women volunteer staff members.	<u>Intervention</u> Memory wallet intervention was designed to improve social participation. Memory wallets were created by volunteers with support/cooperation of family members, after training with the investigator. <u>Outcome Measures</u> Outcome measures were client behaviors and volunteer behaviors coded on the basis of transcriptions of verbal conversations between clients and volunteers. Volunteers and family members completed a satisfaction rating form after the intervention was complete.	When clients were given their memory wallets, the number of factual statements increased from baseline. All clients reduced their use of ambiguous statements during intervention; clients had varying outcomes in response to the intervention in unintelligible, perseverative, or error utterances. Volunteers' use of prompts either maintained or decreased during the intervention; using statements was variable across clients; asking questions decreased slightly for 2 clients and markedly for 2. Volunteers and family members reported satisfaction with communication after introduction of the memory wallet intervention.	The small sample size of clients and volunteers limited data analyses and generalizability. One client seemed less responsive to the intervention, which may have been linked to cognitive status. Future research might examine the functional levels of reading and cognition needed to benefit from the intervention. It is not clear if the memory wallet would be useful to support social participation in conversation with anyone other than a designated volunteer who had been involved in creating the wallet.	Memory wallets may be useful to support social participation and conversations for people with dementia who are able to read but who are having difficulty engaging in conversations. Volunteers may be trained to develop the wallets and participate in conversations with clients.

Bourgeois, M. S., & Mason, L. A. (1996). Memory wallet intervention in an adult day-care setting. *Behavioral Interventions, 11,* 3–18.

(continued)

EVIDENCE TABLE: What is the evidence for the effect of interventions designed to establish, modify, and maintain activities of daily living (ADLs), instrumental activities of daily living (IADLs), leisure, and social participation on the quality of life, health and wellness, and client and caregiver satisfaction for persons with dementia? *(continued)*

Author/Year	Study Objectives	Level/Design/ Participants	Intervention and Outcome Measures	Results	Study Limitations	Implications for Occupational Therapy
Brooker & Duce, 2000	The objective was to compare levels of well-being demonstrated by individuals with mild to moderate dementia using 3 types of activity: reminiscence therapy, structured group activity, and unstructured time.	<u>Level IV</u> Descriptive within-participants repeated measures <u>Participants</u> 25 participants of a day hospital in rural UK. People with mild to moderate dementia of the AD or vascular type. Participants were observed in each group setting for 2 sessions of approximately 40 min over 2 consecutive weeks.	<u>Intervention</u> ■ Reminiscence therapy planned around a theme (e.g., famous people, holidays) ■ Structured group—exercise or craft activities ■ Unstructured time—minimal involvement between staff and patients <u>Outcome Measures</u> Dementia Care Mapping used to measure well-being and ill-being	Well-being differed significantly as a function of the type of activity introduced ($p < .0001$). Reminiscence therapy resulted in higher levels of well-being than general activity or unstructured time.	Since each patient experienced all groups, carryover of skills from one condition to another could have resulted. Assessors were not blinded. Study sample was small and group was a rural, close-knit community that shared long and collective memories.	Occupational therapists can assist in developing structured activity and reminiscence therapy at an appropriate level for patient's cognitive ability. This may result in improved well-being and quality of life for patients.

Brooker, D., & Duce, L. (2000). Well-being and activity in dementia: A comparison of group reminiscence therapy, structured goal-directed group activity and unstructured time. *Aging and Mental Health, 4,* 354–358.

| Lai, Chi, & Kayser-Jones, 2004 | The study was designed to answer the following questions:

• Is specific reminiscence adopting a life-story approach a useful intervention for promoting social well-being in people with dementia in nursing homes?

• If it is useful, can its effects be sustained for 6 weeks after the intervention? | Level I
RCT

Participants were randomized to 1 of 3 groups: reminiscence therapy (RT), comparison group (CG), control group (CC).

ITT group $n = 101$
Per protocol group $n = 86$.

Residents of nursing homes with dementia in Hong Kong. | Intervention
Reminiscence therapy = life-story approach to reminiscence—highly focused triggers to stimulate recall during conversation. 30-min sessions, weekly × 6 weeks.

Comparison group = discussions but not related to life experiences

Control group = no intervention

Outcome Measures:
Social Engagement Scale and WIB | No significant differences were found (in either ITT or per protocol groups) when comparing the outcome variables between T-1 and T-0, T-2 and T-1, and T-2 and T-0 for each individual group.

However, within the ITT intervention group there were significant changes noted when comparing T-1 and T-0 WIB and T-2 and T-0 Social Engagement Scale. Since the test for significant changes in WIB score reached a power of 80%, the finding that the intervention did produce significant improvements in the well-being of the participants can be regarded as fairly convincing. | Authors state that the sample was not large enough for repeated measures multivariate analysis.

The dosage may not have been sufficient. Measures may not have been sensitive enough. | The outcomes provide some evidence of a positive effect of reminiscence on WIB that is sustainable over a period of 6 wk. Longer term sustainability is questioned and in fact the authors indicate that the intervention may need to be ongoing. Occupational therapists wishing to use this intervention still need to determine which features of reminiscence and under what circumstances will have greater or lesser benefits. No harm was detected from the intervention, and there may be some patient and caregiver satisfaction in the process that is worth considering. It is relatively easy to implement at little cost and may assist in improving the quality of social interaction between persons with dementia and their caregivers. |

Lai, C. K. Y., Chi, I., & Kayser-Jones, J. (2004). A randomized controlled trial of a specific reminiscence approach to promote the well-being of nursing home residents with dementia. *International Psychogeriatrics, 16,* 33–49.

(continued)

EVIDENCE TABLE: What is the evidence for the effect of interventions designed to establish, modify, and maintain activities of daily living (ADLs), instrumental activities of daily living (IADLs), leisure, and social participation on the quality of life, health and wellness, and client and caregiver satisfaction for persons with dementia? *(continued)*

Author/Year	Study Objectives	Level/Design/ Participants	Intervention and Outcome Measures	Results	Study Limitations	Implications for Occupational Therapy
Wilkinson, Srikumar, Shaw, & Orrell, 1998	The objective was to investigate the effects of drama therapy in a group of older adults with dementia.	Level II 2-group prospective comparison Participants 16 clients of a psychiatric day hospital, all with dementia.	Intervention The intervention group received a drama and movement group intervention for 12 wk, 1.75 hr/wk. Outcome Measure GHQ-12	Intervention group: Mean scores on the GHQ-12 rose from 15.4 to 17.7 at follow-up, indicating deterioration. Control group: mean scores stayed the same at 17.0. p values were not reported.	Control group was made up of people not selected for the drama group; therefore, there was no random allocation to groups. Control and intervention groups appear to be different in gender, and cognitive and functional status. Sample size was quite small, although power analysis was not completed. It is not clear if the control group received similar attention as the drama group.	Considering the limitations, along with the fact that the data do not support the use of the drama therapy group, the results of this study cannot be used to consider implementing such a program for people with dementia.

Wilkinson, N., Srikumar, S., Shaw, K., & Orrell, M. (1998). Drama and movement therapy in dementia: A pilot study. *Arts in Psychotherapy, 25,* 195–201.

Wishart, Macerollo, Loney, King, Beaumont, Browne, et al., 2000	The objective was to evaluate the effectiveness of a volunteer visiting/ walking program on caregiver burden, social support, health care expenditures, and caregiver satisfaction.	Level I RCT Participants 24 people with cognitive impairment, living with a caregiver, who were able to go on outings.	Intervention Trained volunteers visited care recipients weekly for 6 wk; visits included crafts, walking, and conversation. Control: wait list Outcome Measure Caregiver satisfaction	All caregivers rated their satisfaction at good or excellent for 6/8 items on the client satisfaction score. For the other 2 items, 1 caregiver reported fair (met my needs) or poor (satisfied with help). Satisfaction data were reported as descriptive data because there were no control group data.	Satisfaction ratings were specific to the intervention, so only the intervention group caregivers completed the measure once at the end of the 6 wk. The sample size was small. Caregiver and client health outcomes were not evaluated.	From this study, occupational therapists could consider involvement in a volunteer visiting and walking program, because caregivers reported high levels of satisfaction; however, further research or program evaluation is warranted to compare this intervention to other types of volunteer interventions.

Wishart, L., Macerollo, J., Loney, P., King, A., Beaumont, L., Browne, G., et al. (2000). "Special steps": An effective visiting/walking program for persons with cognitive impairment. *Canadian Journal of Nursing Research, 31,* 57–71.

EVIDENCE TABLE: What is the evidence for the effect of interventions designed to modify and maintain perceptual abilities on the occupational performance of people with dementia?

Author/Year	Study Objectives	Level/Design/ Participants	Intervention and Outcome Measures	Results	Study Limitations	Implications for Occupational Therapy
Interventions that aim to change perception						
Baillon, van Diepen, Prettyman, Redman, Rooke, & Campbell, 2004	The objective was to study the value of Snoezelen on the agitated behavior of people with dementia using a comparison intervention (reminiscence) to control for the effects of increased staff attention. Baillon et al., 2005, reported on individual responses from the same study, whereas this study reported on differences between groups.	Level I Randomized, controlled, crossover design Participants 25 participants recruited from 2 units of care for older people with mental health problems (primarily in the day hospitals) and 1 charity-run nursing home Inclusion criteria: Diagnosis of dementia. Rated by staff as having significant agitation.	Intervention 1-to-1 Snoezelen intervention and reminiscence intervention were provided by trained staff members at the respective units for three 40-min sessions over 2 wk. Outcome Measures ■ Agitation Behavior Mapping Instrument (AMBI) ■ Heart rate monitor ■ Interact Short scale (modified)	There was no statistically significant difference between Snoezelen and reminiscence sessions in level of agitation from presession to immediately postsession ($p = .18$), nor from presession to 15 min postsession ($p = .87$). There was no significant difference between the 2 interventions in the number of items on the Interact Scale showing positive change during the session ($p = .11$) or negative change during the session ($p = .88$).	Power analysis based on data from a pilot study was used to determine that 16 people per group would be adequate to detect a change of 3 points on the main outcome (ABMI). However, the responses were very heterogeneous and both groups improved, suggesting that a larger sample size may be required to detect a difference, if one exists. Potential participants were identified by staff, which could indicate bias of selecting participants most likely to benefit.	Snoezelen had positive results in reducing agitation and improving mood and behaviors, but not significantly more than reminiscence. Of the two interventions, only Snoezelen targets perception. Communication was the only occupational performance outcome measured and is not discussed in the results of this paper. Evidence from this study could not be used to justify its purchase. However, it may be worthwhile to implement on a trial basis with clients with dementia in settings with Snoezelen equipment.

Baillon, S., van Diepen, E., Prettyman, R., Redman, J., Rooke, N., & Campbell, R. (2004). Comparison of the effects of Snoezelen and reminiscence therapy on the agitated behaviour of patients with dementia. *International Journal of Geriatric Psychiatry, 19*, 1047–1052.

(continued)

EVIDENCE TABLE: What is the evidence for the effect of interventions designed to modify and maintain perceptual abilities on the occupational performance of people with dementia? (continued)

Author/Year	Study Objectives	Level/Design/ Participants	Intervention and Outcome Measures	Results	Study Limitations	Implications for Occupational Therapy
Baillon, van Diepen, Prettyman, Rooke, Redman, & Campbell, 2005	The objective was to study the impact of Snoezelen on agitated behavior of people with dementia using a comparison intervention (reminiscence) to control for the effects of increased staff attention. Baillon et al, 2004, reported on group differences from the same study, whereas this report focused on individual responses of participants.	<u>Level I</u> Randomized, controlled, crossover design <u>Participants</u> 25 participants with a diagnosis of dementia and rated by staff in a day hospital and nursing home as having significant agitation were included in the study. *Inclusion criteria:* Diagnosis of dementia. Rated by staff as having significant agitation.	<u>Intervention</u> 1-to-1 Snoezelen intervention and reminiscence intervention were provided by trained staff members at the respective units for three 40-min sessions over 2 wk <u>Outcome Measures</u> ▪ AMBI ▪ Heart rate monitor ▪ Interact Short scale (modified)	The results of the individual responses demonstrated highly variable responses. Snoezelen resulted in more positive mood and behavior ratings than reminiscence for those with severe dementia. These participants had a significantly higher number of items with a positive change on the Interact scale for the Snoezelen session ($p = .01$) compared with reminiscence. There were no differences between the two interventions for agitated behaviors or heart rate.	Power analysis based on data from a pilot study was used to determine that 16 people per group would be adequate to detect a change of 3 points on the main outcome (ABMI). However, the responses were very heterogeneous and both groups improved, suggesting a larger sample size may be required to detect a difference, if one exists. Potential participants were identified by staff, which could indicate bias of selecting participants most likely to benefit.	The variable responses of individuals suggest that trial and caution may be needed in determining who is likely to benefit. People with severe dementia had more positive outcomes in terms of mood and behavior, which may be related to the language demands of reminiscence that are not equivalent with Snoezelen.

Baillon, S., van Diepen, E., Prettyman, R., Rooke, N., Redman, J., & Campbell, R. (2005). Variability in response to older people with dementia to both Snoezelen and reminiscence. *British Journal of Occupational Therapy, 68,* 367–374.

| Baker, Bell, Baker, Gibson, Holloway, Pearce, et al., 2001 | The objective was to evaluate the immediate effects of multisensory stimulation, the carryover effects on behavior and mood in a day hospital and at home, and the endurance of any changes once the sessions have stopped, in comparison with a control condition (activity sessions). | Level I
RCT

Participants
N = 50

Inclusion criteria:
- Living at home with a primary carer
- Referral to the Elderly Mental Health Service of Dorset Health Care NHS Trust by general practitioner
- Consultant psychiatrist's diagnosis of either AD, vascular, or mixed dementia, as recorded in medical notes and corroborated by the research assistant using items from the CANDEX diagnostic
- Attendance at 1 of the 3 day centers on 2 or more days a week.

There were baseline differences between the groups in MMSE and REHAB Deviant Behavior scores. | Intervention
The group of participants in the multisensory stimulation group received 2 sessions of multisensory stimulation per week for 4 wk. The activity group was engaged in activity for the same period of time. Both interventions were delivered by a key worker.

Outcome Measures:
- INTERACT Short
- INTERACT 22-item
- REHAB
- BMD
- BRS | Immediate Effects: Multisensory Stimulation Group had a greater increase in attentiveness to their environment after session ($p = .03$)

Within Session Effects: Patients interacted appropriately with objects more of the time in the activity sessions than in the multisensory stimulation sessions ($p = .001$).

Carryover effects to other environments:

3 significant interaction effects were noted:
1. At the day hospital: The Activity Group improved on the REHAB Speech Subscale over the 4-wk trial period ($p = .037$ after adjusting for group differences).
2. At home: Multisensory Stimulation Group improved on the BMD scale total score and BRS social disturbance subscale. The Activity Group deteriorated over the course of the sessions in the BMD scale total score and showed no changes in the BRS social disturbance subscale. When these differences were tested adjusting for baseline group differences, the difference in social disturbance scores was not statistically significant; the difference in BMD Scale total score had a p value of .051. | It is not clear whether the individuals who administered the assessments also administered the intervention.

Psychometric properties of the outcome measures are not reported.

Sample size is not justified.

It is unclear whether the participants received any other intervention in addition to the study. | On the basis of the results from this study, it appears that multisensory stimulation and activity-based sessions were overall well received in terms of mood and behaviors. Speech skills were the only occupational performance outcome evaluated; the Activity Group improved more during the 4-wk sessions than the multisensory stimulation group. The findings indicate a beneficial effect of structured 1-to-1 activities. It is not clear that these activities sessions targeted perception. |

(continued)

Author/Year	Study Objectives	Level/Design/ Participants	Intervention and Outcome Measures	Results	Study Limitations	Implications for Occupational Therapy
Baker, Bell, Baker, Gibson, Holloway, Pearce et al., 2001 *(cont.)*				*Follow up:* On the BMD total score, the Multisensory Stimulation Group lost any improvement they had gained in behavior during the trial and demonstrated a significant deterioration at the 1 mo follow-up.		

Baker, R., Bell, S., Baker, E., Gibson, S., Holloway, J., & Pearce, R., et al. (2001). A randomized controlled trial of the effects of multi-sensory stimulation (MSS) for people with dementia. *British Journal of Clinical Psychology, 40,* 81–96.

Author/Year	Study Objectives	Level/Design/ Participants	Intervention and Outcome Measures	Results	Study Limitations	Implications for Occupational Therapy
Baker, Dowling, Wareing, Dawson, & Assey, 1997	The objective was to investigate the long-term and short-term effects of the Snoezelen environment on the behavior, mood, and cognition of elderly patients with dementia, as well as to gain an understanding of the processes occurring within Snoezelen.	Level I RCT Participants 36 participants who met the inclusion criteria were included in the study. *Inclusion criteria:* • Diagnosed with Alzheimer's disease or vascular dementia • Referred to the Elderly Severely Mentally III Service of the Dorset HealthCare NHS Trust by a general practitioner • Living at home with a main caregiver • Attended 1 of 2 day hospitals within the Trust twice a week or more	Intervention Participants in Group 1 received Snoezelen intervention (nondirective) twice a week for 4 wk. Participants in Group II received directed activity sessions twice a week for 4 wk. Outcome Measures • REHAB • BMD • BRS, part of the CAPE • Mini-mental state exam • CAS, part of the CAPE • Interact	Participants in the Snoezelen group changed little in REHAB deviant behavior scores, whereas the activity group participants had significantly higher scores ($p < .01$), indicating worse behavior). Caregiver ratings of social disturbance indicated significantly better behavior in the Snoezelen group and worse behavior in the activity group ($p < .005$). REHAB speech scores improved for the Snoezelen group from pretrial to posttrial, but they decreased at follow-up. In the activity group, speech skills deteriorated from pretrial to posttrial, but improved again at follow-up. Short-term results indicated improvement in 8 of 12 behavior and mood rating items (including doing things on own initiative, talking spontaneously), but the improvement was the same in both groups.	Minimal information is provided about the psychometrics of the measures, making it difficult to ensure appropriate outcome measures. Sample size was not justified on the basis of a power analysis, and no post hoc power analysis was reported. While exact *p* values were not reported, the baseline differences between groups and the multiple analyses may have resulted in errors.	The short-term effects of Snoezelen compared with an activity intervention do not demonstrate either to be more effective than the other. The long-term effects 1 mo postintervention may suggest that Snoezelen had positive impacts on socially disturbed behaviors. The results do not justify the benefits of investing in Snoezelen equipment in a hospital or nursing home. It would be beneficial for future research to examine outcomes longer than 1 mo postintervention, and importantly to occupational therapy, to link any behavioral outcomes to occupational performance outcomes.

Baker, R., Dowling, Z., Wareing, L. A., Dawson, J., & Assey, J. (1997). Snoezelen: Its long-term and short-term effects on older people with dementia. *British Journal of Occupational Therapy, 60,* 213–218.

| Chung & Lai, 2002 | The objective was to review the clinical efficacy of Snoezelen for older people with dementia. | Level I Systematic review RCTs in which Snoezelen or multisensory programs were used as an intervention for people with dementia (any type) age > 60. | N/A | 2 RCTs were included in the analysis.

1. Parallel group design, 50 participants
2. Randomized crossover design with 17 participants

The search was updated in 2004 with no new RCTs identified.

Outcomes sometime after treatment sessions (4 & 8 sessions): There were no differences between treatment and control groups on most subscores, but 1 was significant after 4 sessions. After 8 sessions, 4 subscores were statistically significant, including speech skills ($p = .03$).

Immediately after treatment sessions and at 1 mo follow-up (long-term effects), no significant differences were identified. | N/A | This systematic review found limited evidence to support or refute the use of Snoezelen in clinical practice with people with dementia. The therapeutic value of this intervention in relation to occupational performance outcomes has not been established through this systematic review. Although there were no indications of harmful effects from the Snoezelen intervention, there is little to justify the cost or time required to offer the intervention. In settings in which the equipment has already been purchased, Snoezelen may be used with adults with dementia if they seem to enjoy the experience. |

Chung, J. C. C., & Lai, C. K. Y. (2002). Snoezelen for dementia. *Cochrane Database of Systematic Reviews*, Issue 4. Art. No.: CD003152. DOI: 10.1002/1565 1858.CD003152.

(continued)

Author/Year	Study Objectives	Level/Design/ Participants	Intervention and Outcome Measures	Results	Study Limitations	Implications for Occupational Therapy
Heyn, 2003	The objective was to evaluate the outcomes of a multisensory exercise program on cognitive function, behavior, and physiological indexes in 13 nursing home residents diagnosed with moderate to severe Alzheimer's disease.	Level III 1 group, pretest– posttest design Participants A convenience sample of 13 participants who met the inclusion criteria (.65, diagnosis of dementia, have mobility, < 21 on MMSE)	Intervention Multisensory exercise program with 4 components: ■ Focused attention and warm-up session ■ Flexibility and aerobic exercises ■ Strength training session ■ Session closure Provided by an exercise physiologist 3×/wk for 8 wk Nursing staff asked to report any significant changes in medica- tion, diet, schedule, and activities. Outcome Measures ■ Menorah Park Engagement Scale ■ Resting heart rate ■ Blood pressure ■ Weight ■ Caregiver Mood Report	*Engagement*: Engagement improved from before to after intervention with 9 of 13 participants engaged in more than half of the activity. *Mood*: 8 participants showed positive improvements in overall mood; 5 showed no signif- icant or little improvement. *Resting heart rate*: Mean heart rate improved significantly ($p = .01$). *Blood pressure and weight*: No significant change was reported. The author states that "preliminary findings sug- gest that multisensory exercise approaches may decrease RHR, increase exercise engagement and preserve function in per- sons with AD" (p. 250).	Limitations include the following: ■ Lack of comparison group ■ A small convenience sample ■ Multiple outcome measures, including some with question- able psychometric properties Limitations make it difficult to draw conclusions about the value of a multisensory exercise program. Conclusion about preservation of function is not valid because it was not one of the outcome measures used.	As the authors correctly discuss, it can be challenging to engage people with dementia in physical activity programs. This program is of inter- est because it draws on a multisensory approach, including using perceptual components to engage people in a physical activity program. Further evidence is needed to demonstrate that a multisensory approach is a useful means to engage people in such a physi- cal activity program, and that it results in functional gains as well.

Heyn, P. (2003). The effect of a multisensory exercise program on engagement, behavior, and selected physiological indexes in persons with dementia. *American Journal of Alzheimer's Disease and Other Dementias, 18*, 247–251.

| Hope, 1998 | The objective was to determine how older people with dementia respond to the individual pieces of equipment in the multisensory room and to examine the extent to which exposure to the room influenced the observed behavior of patients both in the short and medium term. | Level III Descriptive study Participants 29 participants with a diagnosis of dementia, experiencing the multisensory room as part of their ongoing care | Intervention Frequency and duration: 45 sessions over an 8-mo period. Amount of sessions per patient varied from 1 to 4 sessions. Individual sessions varied in duration: 30 min or more, or 20 min or more. 21 staff members were given instructions on the use of the equipment and a written protocol was developed. Outcome Measures An assessment package was completed at each session by the accompanying staff member. It included the following: ■ Demographic data ■ Information about behavior observed before and after the session ■ Patient's response to individual pieces of equipment ■ Patient's response in the room—using the Interact ■ Pulse rate measurements before and after sessions | Results were not reported in terms of statistical significance. 55% of the patients demonstrated a negative response to the equipment. Of 21 patients who had any negative response, 13 patients had an overall positive score. 35.6% (n = 16) associated with higher levels of happiness and contentment. 22.2% and less fear and anxiety. Spontaneity of speech increased on 7 occasions (15.6%); sensibility of speech increased over the session on 5 instances. Eye contact improved in 11 sessions. Stimulation (4 conditions): ■ Undesirably active: For n = 25 none. On 16 occasions when this activity did occur, it was reported to have, < over the session on 6 and > on 3. ■ Desirably active: For n = 8 none. In 23 of 45 sessions it was evident some of the time. It increased in 12 sessions (26.7%). | Sample size was not justified. Psychometric properties of the outcome measure were not stated in this study. Multiple staff members were involved in carrying out the intervention. There was a lack of standardization of intervention, despite protocol. There were issues with interrater reliability. The assessment method lacks rigor. The authors did not control for variability in diagnosis of dementia. Given these limitations, care should be taken when interpreting the results of this study, particularly given the high cost generally associated with the creation of multisensory rooms. | Study results favor the use of multisensory sessions for people with dementia, particularly with low mood or anxiety; however, a positive experience did not occur for all patients, particularly around the tactile equipment. Further, the level of evidence and quality of the evidence suggests the conclusion should be interpreted with caution. The variable responses suggest the need for client-centered approaches and care plans. Program development needs to include education, rationale for the intervention, organization of the implementation, and maintaining motivation. The study does not provide strong support for implementing a multisensory room if one does not already exist. |

(continued)

EVIDENCE TABLE: What is the evidence for the effect of interventions designed to modify and maintain perceptual abilities on the occupational performance of people with dementia? (continued)

Author/Year	Study Objectives	Level/Design/ Participants	Intervention and Outcome Measures	Results	Study Limitations	Implications for Occupational Therapy
Hope, 1998 *(cont.)*			▪ Summary of the per- ceived effect on the pa- tient from the member of staff's perspective	▪ Undesirably inactive: $n = 29$ sessions (64.4%) —absent. ▪ Desirably inactive: 75.5% of the patients were judged to be appropriately relaxed and desirable inactivity increased in 11 cases (24.4%). Pulse rate: No significant difference were reported in before and after sessions.		

Hope, K. (1998). The effects of multisensory environments on older people with dementia. *Journal of Psychiatric and Mental Health Nursing, 5,* 377–385.

| Lantz, Buchalter, & McBee, 1997 | The objective was to describe a group designed to build on residents' strengths by enhancing residents' self-awareness. The study also reported on the initial evaluation of this group. | **Level II**
 2-group, nonrandomized study (Level II) and case studies (Level V).

 Participants
 14 participants with a diagnosis of dementia were selected on the basis of their atten- dance in the interven- tion group program. No other inclusion criteria were reported. | **Intervention**
 Group 1: 8–10 residents grouped by cognitive status and severity of dementia met weekly for 1 hr for 10 wk. Intervention was delivered by a phys- iatrist and social worker. The group program focused on modified meditation, relaxation, guided imagery, and body awareness.

 Group 2: Received usual care and no specific intervention.

 Outcome Measures
 CMAI | CMAI scores for intervention group: Median change was −15.5 (range −32.0 to −4.0), SD = 10.4 ($p < .001$). The median change for the Control Group was −1.0 (range −2.0 to +2.0) SD = 1.6 ($p \leq .001$). Both groups showed improvement, although the Intervention Group showed greater reductions in agitation.

 Case vignettes demonstrate that the group was useful in reducing physical aggressiveness, helping a resident cope with increasing frailty, and offering an alternative to verbal disruption. | Staff became aware of techniques and group membership and were spontaneously using the same in their daily work. Therefore, not necessarily confined to intervention group.

 It is not known whether the intervention is respon- sible for the change in resident behavior or perhaps another factor. The level of evi- dence is very low and suggests that more study is required. | The theoretical constructs of this study are client centered and empower- ing, and it has potential to be within the scope of occupational therapy practice as an intervention using perceptual skills and cognitive skills to change behavior. Further evaluation is recom- mended with more strin- gent examination before its inclusion as a possible intervention for clients with dementia. |

Lantz, M. S., Buchalter, E. N., & McBee, L. (1997). Wellness group: A novel intervention for coping with disruptive behavior in elderly nursing home residents. *Gerontologist, 37,* 551–556.

| Pinkney, 1997 | The objective was to compare the effectiveness of the Snoezelen environment to a relaxation technique (music) in manipulating mood and behavior in patients with senile dementia. | Level IV

Single-case design (3 cases) ABC design where A = baseline, B = Snoezelen, C = music

Participants

3 participants attending a day program and who met the inclusion criteria were enrolled in the study. | Intervention

Participants observed in day hospital setting, by an occupational therapist 3×/wk for 3 wk. Observations made at 1-min intervals for 30 min.

A (baseline): Each participant was alone and observed sitting in an armchair with no extra stimulation.

B (Snoezelen): Each participant was alone and observed sitting in an armchair in Snoezelen environment.

C (music relaxation group): 6 participants were observed seated in armchairs, listening to classical music selected by their care providers.

Outcome Measures

Assessment of short-term manipulation of affect in severely demented. | Case 1: Improvements noted in mood and behavior in response to both interventions.

Case 2: Improvements noted in mood and behavior in both treatment settings. Singing increased in music setting.

Case 3: Observations of behavior fluctuated dramatically throughout baseline and the treatment sessions, with a particular increase in movement and level of happiness. Snoezelen caused higher incidence of happiness and looking.

Following descriptive information about the responses of each of the participants, the authors noted that Snoezelen and music are equally effective in manipulating mood and affect in a positive way. Each media can be used to stimulate certain responses. Music was better for reminiscence and musical memory. Snoezelen was better for global stimulation and absorbed concentration. | The outcome measure is not commonly used and its validity is not reported. There is a possible intervention bias because participants also received occupational therapy during the study.

While the study is described as a single-case design, each intervention was only introduced once. | Results of the study suggest that Snoezelen and music may be equally effective. Music therapy is less costly and easier to implement. If both interventions assist with increasing positive behavior and mood, then they might be strategies to relieve caregivers for periods of respite time. There is little evidence from this study to suggest that they influence occupational performance in any way. The study is not strong enough to support either intervention. |

Pinkney, L. (1997). A comparison of the Snoezelen environment and a music relaxation group on the mood and behaviour of patients with senile dementia. *British Journal of Occupational Therapy, 60,* 209–212.

(continued)

Author/Year	Study Objectives	Level/Design/ Participants	Intervention and Outcome Measures	Results	Study Limitations	Implications for Occupational Therapy
Pomeroy, 1993	The objective was to assess whether providing a physiotherapy intervention improves or maintains the mobility skills of elderly people with a severe dementing illness.	Level I Randomized crossover. Patients were randomly allocated to physiotreatment followed by no-treatment phase or vice versa. Participants 24 participants who met the inclusion criteria were included in the study.	Intervention Control group received no intervention for 6 wk. Physiotreatment group received music and movement, body awareness, and individual functional/mobility training (three 30-min sessions per week for 6 wk). Outcome Measures Southampton Assessment of Mobility	There was wide variation in individual mobility scores, but results indicated improved mobility scores during the treatment phase and decreased mobility during the control phase. Statistical analyses of changes in mobility scores between treatment and control phases indicated a probable treatment effect $-.05 > p > .01$ (Wilcoxon signed ranks test).	Study does not address long-term effect of intervention (i.e., are gains maintained?). Relatively high rate of noncompletion (33%) may be a result of natural progression of the disease or an indication that the intervention was too strenuous.	Study demonstrates that even people with severe cognitive impairment can benefit from the intervention that focused on body awareness, movement, and mobility.

Pomeroy, V. M. (1993). The effect of physiotherapy input on mobility skills of elderly people with severe dementing illness. *Clinical Rehabilitation, 7,* 163–170.

Robichaud, Hebert, & Desrosiers, 1994	The objective was to verify whether a sensory integration program improves the behavior and functioning of institutionalized patients with dementia.	Level I RCT Participants 40 participants Inclusion criteria: Age ≥ 60; fulfilled the DSM-III-R criteria for dementia; scored < 75 (out of 100) on the Modified MMSE; had > 1 disruptive behavior; and were physically able to attend the sessions	Intervention Sensory integration group: Three 45-min standardized sensory integration sessions per week for 10 wk in 3 different institutional settings. The intervention was conducted in a room close to care units following the 5 steps set out by Ross and Budick. Control group: Participants participated in leisure activities at their respective institutions for 10 wk. Limited information provided about the duration of sessions. Outcome Measures ■ Revised Memory and Behavior Problem Checklist ■ Psycho Geriatric Scale of Basic Activities of Daily Living	Treatment Group: There was a decrease in frequency of disruptive behaviors ($t = 3.16$, $p = .004$); decrease of the caregivers' reaction to behaviors ($t = 5.80$, $p = .0001$); an improvement in ADLs ($t = 2.91$, $p = .009$). Control Group: The control group exhibited similar changes but these were not statistically significant except for the reaction to the disruptive behavior ($t = 2.15$, $p = .05$). ANCOVA: The intervention had no significant effect on the behaviors of the treatment group compared to the control.	There was questionable power and limited scope and sensitivity of outcome measures. There may have been contamination because of the study design. The authors report that frequency of sessions may not have been frequent enough. The stage of dementia may have been irreversible and therefore may have contributed to the lack of ability to verify efficacy of SI programs.	The idea for using sensory stimulation for people with dementia is sound, and the concept of the activities is within the scope of occupational therapy practice. The authors noted several limitations of the study: contamination effect on caregiver attitudes, frequency of sessions (may not have been frequent enough), small sample size, the need to consider other outcome measures, stage of dementia. They recommend further studies be done. However, this study does not provide evidence of the effectiveness of sensory integration.

Robichaud, L., Hebert, R., & Desrosiers, J. (1994). Efficacy of a sensory integration program on behaviors of inpatients with dementia. *American Journal of Occupational Therapy, 48,* 355–360.

Citation	Objective	Level/Design/Participants	Intervention/Outcome Measures	Results	Comments
Rosswurm, 1990	The objective was to investigate the effectiveness of an AFG program as an intervention for stimulating the perceptual–cognitive processing, functional performance, and social interactions of persons with dementia.	Level I RCT (pretest–posttest control group design) Participants 30 participants selected from 3 skilled nursing homes Inclusion criteria: Diagnosis of dementia of the AD or multi-infarct types; < 20 on the Folstein MMSE	Intervention Group I (AFG): 3 activity segments: Welcoming and relaxation exercises; perceptual-matching exercises; reinforcement with refreshments Group II: Social interaction and refreshments but no planned program Frequency: 30 min 3 times/wk for 4 wk Outcome Measures ■ Dementia Behavior Scale ■ MMSE ■ Perceptual-matching tasks ■ Check sheets	Significant improvements: Participation in AFGs resulted in improved performance of the visual-matching exercises and group activities ($p <$ .001). Statistically significant improvements in the perceptual processing of information and in the social interactions of persons who participated in the AFG did not transfer to functional performance, particularly psychomotor skills needed for ADLs.	Sample size was not justified. There was a potential for sample selection bias. The restrictive nature of the nursing home on independent performance, changes in health status, brevity of the intervention, and the lack of sensitive functional assessment tools may have influenced the lack of impact on functional outcome. Future studies should trace all such impacting variables.	Use of an attention-focusing program with persons with advanced dementia is worth further investigation and consideration. Statistically significant improvements in the person's ability to improve perceptual processing of information and social interaction in the AFG are encouraging and suggest that persons with advanced dementia can learn to compensate for perceptual processing deficits, if only to a limited degree.

Rosswurm, M. A. (1990). Attention-focusing program for persons with dementia. *Clinical Gerontologist, 10*, 3–16.

Citation	Objective	Level/Design/Participants	Intervention/Outcome Measures	Results	Comments
Sherratt, Thornton, & Hatton, 2004	The objective was to determine whether there were differences in responses of people with dementia to a live music condition compared to recorded music conditions and a no music condition.	Level III An experimental, within-participants, repeated measures design Participants $N = 24$ Inclusion criteria: ■ Formal diagnosis of dementia ■ Moderate to severe level of cognitive impairment ■ History of challenging behavior or signs of social withdrawal and minimal engagement	Intervention participants with similar music preferences were divided into 5 groups of ≤ 8 people. All music conditions were provided for 1 hr. Responses of participants to no music, commercially recorded music, recorded music by musician, and live music condition were observed. Outcome Measures Using continuous time sampling, nonparticipant observational data were collected.	Recorded and live music appear to be effective in decreasing the amount of time spent engaged in meaningless activity or sleeping; live music was found to be more beneficial. Recorded and live music were effective in increasing levels of well-being/extreme well-being when compared to the no-music condition; and live music was the most effective method.	The validity of the outcome measures are not reported in the article.	Through the use of music, engagement in meaningful activity can be increased. This can be implemented for older adults who are cared for in nursing homes who are diagnosed with moderate to severe cognitive impairments. By engaging in meaningful activity, a feeling of well-being can result. This in turn may affect quality of life.

Sherratt, K., Thornton, A., & Hatton, C. (2004). Emotional and behavioural responses to music in people with dementia: An observational study. *Aging and Mental Health, 8*, 233–241.

(continued)

EVICENCE TABLE: What is the evidence for the effect of interventions designed to modify and maintain perceptual abilities on the occupational performance of people with dementia? (continued)

Author/Year	Study Objectives	Level/Design/Participants	Intervention and Outcome Measures	Results	Study Limitations	Implications for Occupational Therapy
van Diepen, Baillon, Redman, Rooke, Spencer, & Prettyman, 2002	The objective was to evaluate the feasibility of using a detailed approach to behavioral and physiological assessments before, during, and after Snoezelen sessions for patients with various forms of dementia. In addition, the objective was to identify whether there were any large effects of the intervention that might be relevant in refining the methodology for a definitive study.	Level I RCT pilot study Participants 15 participants recruited from a psychiatry day hospital program for elderly people and 1 participant recruited from an acute organic assessment ward. 2 study groups: 1 received Snoezelen therapy and the other received reminiscence therapy. Significant differences within groups in terms of severity of dementia and degree of cognitive impairment at baseline.	Intervention Intervention group (n = 8): 8 individual Snoezelen sessions in a specially designed multisensory room. Comparison group: 8 individual reminiscence therapy sessions in a separate room in the facility. Both sessions were 40 min, 2×/wk for 4 wk Outcome Measures ■ Short form of the CMAI ■ ABMI ■ The Interact Scale	CMAI: After 4 wk and at follow-up, both groups had a tendency for lower scores (not statistically significant). ABMI: Snoezelen group had a lower score immediately after the session but not sustained 15 and 30 min after intervention. The reminiscence group increased score over the 4 time points (not statistically significant). Interact scale: Both groups indicate a positive outcome on participants' behavior and occasional negative outcome.	Sample size (n = 15) was not large enough to show a difference statistically. The groups were not homogenous; therefore, analyses of a descriptive nature had to be reported.	There is inadequate evidence on the effects of Snoezelen on agitated behavior and further evidence is required to inform health care providers of the benefits of the same. This pilot study suggests it is possible to recruit people to conduct further research on Snoezelen and suggests that the measures used to examine the effects of Snoezelen on agitated behavior may need to be modified.

van Diepen, E., Baillon, S. F., Redman, J., Rooke, N., Spencer, D. A., & Prettyman, R. (2002). A pilot study of the physiological and behavioural effects of snoezelen in dementia. *British Journal of Occupational Therapy, 65,* 61–66.

Interventions that use remaining perceptual abilities (compensation) but do not change perception

Cohen-Mansfield & Werner, 1998	The objective was to assess the effects of an enhanced environment, as a global variable, on behavior and mood, as well as on the manifestation of pacing and wandering behaviors, of nursing home residents with dementia who pace frequently.	Level IV Multiple single participant (AB) design Participants 27 residents in 1 of 2 buildings, with relatively equivalent hallways, in a large, suburban, nonprofit nursing home who were rated by nursing staff as pacing or wandering several times a day on the pacing item of the CMAI were enrolled in the study.	Intervention Intervention 1 was a nature scene and Intervention 2 was a home and people scene. Each was installed in a nursing home corridor with 2 benches facing the scene to allow people to sit and look at the murals. Intervention 3 was a no stimuli situation—a standard nursing home corridor. Participants were exposed to the interventions for 2 wk, and the research assistant and nursing staff monitored the resident's reactions to the scene. Outcome Measures ■ The Observer, Version 3.0, a handheld computer event recorder ■ Photoelectronic counter ■ Strip-switch counter/time ■ Observational measurement on the computer event recorder ■ Body position ■ Lawton's Modified–Behavior Stream ■ The Confusion Inventory ■ Personal Activity Monitor2 attached at the ankle, detects body movements ■ CMAI, 7-point scale	Residents spent significantly more time in corridors once they were enhanced ($p < .01$) and spent decreased time in other locations (with the exception of the dining room). In the enhanced corridor, residents sat on hallway benches for longer and data from photoelectric counters showed that people used the corridor more; however, the counter counted all people, not just study participants. In simulated corridors, residents sat more and engaged in less exit-seeking and trespassing behavior. Statistical significance was not reached. No statistical significance was noted with pacing behavior. A decrease was observed for most types of agitated behavior when the scenes were on; however, it was not statistically significant. Nurses' ratings reported decreases in aggressive and nonaggressive physical behaviors and in verbally aggressive behaviors; however, it was not statistically significant.	Results should be considered preliminary because multiple analyses were run without controlling for the risk of reaching significance by chance. Staff were not blinded in the study. The intervention is multifaceted, making it difficult to ascertain which parts of the intervention are most effective (e.g., olfactory, visual, tactile, auditory stimulation). The positive effect of the enhanced environment had on staff should not be discounted, but the indirect benefit to residents requires some measurement.	Based solely on this study, it would be difficult to recommend this as an evidence-based intervention. Given the low cost and ease of implementing any part of these simulated environments, as well as the low potential for it causing any harm, it would not be unreasonable to consider these changes in institutions for cognitively impaired residents. However, given the preliminary nature of this study, it would be beneficial to obtain more objective support.

Cohen-Mansfield, J., & Werner, P. (1998). The effects of an enhanced environment on nursing home residents who pace. *Gerontologist, 38*, 199–208.

(continued)

EVIDENCE TABLE: What is the evidence for the effect of interventions designed to modify and maintain perceptual abilities on the occupational performance of people with dementia? (continued)

Author/Year	Study Objectives	Level/Design/ Participants	Intervention and Outcome Measures	Results	Study Limitations	Implications for Occupational Therapy
Dickinson, McLain-Kark, & Marshall-Baker, 1995	The objective was to evaluate the use of a blind and cloth barrier to reduce the attempts to exit on a dementia care unit.	Level III Nonrandomized before–after study design Participants 7 residents on a special care dementia unit that triggered the alarm during the initial observation period	Intervention Week 1: Participants were observed daily to identify a baseline number of exit attempts and which participants would attempt to escape. Week 2: A closed mini-blind was installed covering the window panel or glazing at the doors. Week 4: A cloth barrier was installed with the blind left open. Week 6: Both cloth barrier and blinds were installed. Weeks 3 & 5: No intervention was done; no measurement was taken. Outcome Measures Observers' count and notes on behaviors during the week of intervention.	Activation totals Baseline: 115 times Intervention 1–Closed Blind: 64 attempts (44% decrease) Intervention 2–Panel: 5 attempts (96% decrease) Intervention 3–Closed Blind + Panel: 14 attempts (88% decrease) Wilcoxon rank sum analysis: Intervention 1–Closed Blind: Marginally significant (rank sum = .07, .04 < p < .07) Intervention 2–Panel: Statistically significant (rank sum = 15.5, p < .001) Intervention 3–Panel + Closed Blind: Statistically significant (rank sum = 11, p < .01)	Limited time period of measurement of interventions may have showed initial change as significant but did not allow for time to see whether familiarity would have increased exit attempts due to exploration or learning. Authors believed that residents may have had the capability to learn that the panic bar was behind the visual barrier.	Occupational therapists can recommend environmental changes as a short-term solution to prevent wandering and reduce risk of injury. This intervention has the potential to affect health care delivery in terms of cost, if the need for constant monitoring is reduced by the environmental change. Further investigation is required to determine whether a visual barrier is an effective long-term solution and to determine the type of visual barriers that are most effective at decreasing awareness of exit doors.

Dickinson, J. I., McLain-Kark, J., & Marshall-Baker, A. (1995). The effects of visual barriers on exiting behavior in a dementia care unit. *Gerontologist, 35,* 127–130.

| Elmståhl, Annerstedt, & Åhlund, 1997 | The objective of the study was to evaluate the influence of the design of group living units on behavioral reactions in demented elderly patients. | Level II Cohort study

Participants
105 participants with dementia living in group living units in Sweden

3 groups of variable sizes on the basis of the floor plan of the units at the center | Intervention
Group A: 66 participants (corridor-like designs)
Group B: 8 participants (L-shaped unit)
Group C: 31 participants (square or H shaped design)

The participants in the groups were observed at 3 points over the study period.

Outcome Measures
■ OBS scale
■ Therapeutic Environment Screen Scale
■ Berger scale
■ Katz Index of ADLs
■ MMSE | At 6 mo: Group B had lower time disorientation than Group A ($p < .05$). At 12 mo: Group A had significant reductions (within group) in identity ($p < .05$), whereas the other 2 groups did not have similar reductions (between groups' differences not statistically significant).

Units with ample lighting vs. others: Observed symptoms did not differ. *Amount of space or amount of activity space within a unit:* No differences found in confusional or disorientation symptoms.

Larger communication areas: Associated with less recent memory disorientation ($r = -.16$, $p = .05$), and less time disorientation and less identity disorientation (not statistically significant). | Limited information was provided on the psychometric properties of measures used. There was a small number of residents in Group B, lack of random allocation, and assumed lack of blinding of assessors.

Limitations make it difficult to make definitive conclusions or recommendations related to clinical practice or (floor layout).

It is not clear why the authors have concluded that communication area should not be reduced, because there was no significant difference in the area available for communication and most symptoms of resident | In terms of the occupational performance outcomes from this study (orientation to time and own identity), the results suggest that there may be value in further research on the floor plans of group living units, but definitive conclusions cannot be made. |

Elmståhl, S., Annerstedt, L., & Åhlund, O. (1997). How should a group living unit for demented elderly be designed to decrease psychiatric symptoms? *Alzheimer Disease and Associated Disorders, 11,* 47–52.

(continued)

EVIDENCE TABLE: What is the evidence for the effect of interventions designed to modify and maintain perceptual abilities on the occupational performance of people with dementia? *(continued)*

Author/Year	Study Objectives	Level/Design/ Participants	Intervention and Outcome Measures	Results	Study Limitations	Implications for Occupational Therapy
Gibson, MacLean, Borrie, & Geiger, 2004	The objective was to test the expectation that the majority of residents would be oriented to the location of their own rooms in a new environment, and intrusion into others' rooms would be unintentional and less frequent.	Level IV Descriptive study using systematic observational techniques Participants 19 veterans residing in a dementia care unit	Intervention Members of the health care team oriented residents over an 8-wk interval (using a standardized protocol) after they moved into a new unit. Outcome Measures ▪ Standardized MMSE ▪ Constructional Praxis from the ADAS ▪ Cornell Scale for Depression in Dementia ▪ Intrusion monitoring ▪ Interview of successful residents	Of the study participants, 84% were able to find their own room on initial attempts whereas 16% found their rooms after 3 repetitions of the orientation task. On average, participants reported using cues from 2 of the 4 environmental categories. Thematic analysis of nursing interpretations and residents' comments indicated that a majority of participants who were able to find their own rooms but still intruded other rooms were seeking social interaction.	This study had a small sample size, nonrepresentative sample, and lack of experimental manipulation of variables. Multiple outcomes were analyzed but not analyzed for variance. Perceptual skills level of clients should have been assessed. Data collection and analysis were not clearly reported. Findings and discussion seemed to focus more on reasons for intrusion rather than use of environment for orientation, which was the original purpose of the investigation.	The study suggests further research into how orientation to the environment is affected by social stimulation. A study that measures the use of different perceptual skills for orientation tasks would be beneficial.

Gibson, M. C., MacLean, J., Borrie, M., & Geiger, J. (2004). Orientation behaviors in residents relocated to a redesigned dementia care unit. *American Journal of Alzheimer's Disease and Other Dementias, 19,* 45–49.

Kincaid & Peacock, 2003	The objective was to examine the effect that a wall mural painted over an exit door has on decreasing door-testing behaviors of residents with dementia.	Level III Pretest–posttest Participants A convenience sample of 12 participants Inclusion criteria: Residents of SCU of nursing home, > 65, English speaking, diagnosis of dementia, noncomatose, lived in residence > 2 mo	Intervention On an SCU, a floor-to-ceiling wall mural was painted on the exit door and adjoining walls to disguise doorway. Observations were daily for 6 wks before and 6 wks after mural at a regular 2-hr period 5:30–7:30 pm over 12 wk. Outcome Measures Tally marked door testing behaviors. 4 types of behaviors were observed: ■ Walking up to door and push/pull calmly ■ Waiting for someone to exit and trying to follow them ■ Team effort ■ Exit seeking with force	Total of all types of door testing: Premural door testing 55.67, postmural testing 13.42 ($p = .024$). Type 1 and 3 behaviors decreased most (Type 1 from 35.67 to 6.17, $p < .05$; Type 3 from 3.42 to 0.75, $p < .05$). Type 2 and 4 behaviors decreased, but these were not statistically significant.	It is unclear who observed the behaviors, and there is a timing bias as reporting was done during sundowning.	Although evidence from this study design is not high level, the intervention is low risk and benefits are noted in decreased exit seeking behavior. It appears that the mural had an impact on residents, including decreased exit-seeking behaviors. Further, it is likely that the mural made the environment less institutional.

Kincaid, C., & Peacock, J. R. (2003). Effect of a wall mural on decreasing four types of door-testing behaviors. *Journal of Applied Gerontology, 22*, 76–88.

Koss & Gilmore, 1998	The objective was to test the hypothesis that in sundowning, agitation may be triggered by a decrease in the amount of ambient light available rather than by an internal clock.	Level III Nonrandomized before–after study design Participants A sample of 13 high-functioning residents of the dementia unit of a long-term-care facility, who ate independently	Intervention The intervention consisted of increasing light intensity and enhancing visual stimulation during evening meals. Tables were positioned directly under existing ceiling lights, and were set with settings using maximal visual contrast. Regular nursing home table settings were used at breakfast and lunch. Outcome Measures Food intake record and agitation record were designed for the study; neither have any reported reliability or validity.	The mean amount of food ingested at dinner was significantly higher during intervention than postintervention ($p < .03$). No other paired comparison reached significance. The frequency of agitated behaviors decreased dramatically during the intervention phase $p = .01$. Post hoc analysis showed significant differences in agitation between baseline and intervention ($p < .05$) and between baseline and postintervention ($p < .05$). Further analyses showed that decrease in agitation occurred in the evening $p < .05$ and during the day $p < .1$.	There was no control group or monitoring of other interventions that might have resuited in the observed differences. Measurement instruments were based on staff judgment, with no psychometrics.	The interventions described in this study are strategies familiar to occupational therapists, especially in rehabilitative settings. By recognizing that these same strategies may be beneficial for persons with AD, even in the early stages of the disease, occupational therapists can use these strategies to positively affect the perceptual abilities of this patient population. Although this is a preliminary study, it is worth consideration because it is easy to employ, noninvasive, inexpensive, and poses no risk of harm.

Koss, E., & Gilmore, G. C. (1998). Environmental interventions and functional ability of AD patients. In B. Vellas, J. Fitten, & G. Frisoni (Eds.), *Research and practice in Alzheimer's disease* (pp. 185–193). New York: Springer.

(continued)

Author/Year	Study Objectives	Level/Design/ Participants	Intervention and Outcome Measures	Results	Study Limitations	Implications for Occupational Therapy
McGilton, Rivera, & Dawson, 2003	The objective was to examine the effects of a way-finding intervention on residents' ability to find their way in a new environment.	<u>Level</u> I RCT <u>Participants</u> $n = 32$ nursing home residents 6 wk after relocation to a new facility. Assessments were done at baseline, 1 wk, and 3 mo after intervention. Allocation to a treatment or control group was done randomly after baseline demographics were collected.	<u>Intervention</u> The treatment group received backward chaining involving rehearsal of way-finding; communication techniques to facilitate residents' way-finding; use of an individualized locational map that was delivered by 2 research assistants for 30 min, 3×/wk for 4 wk. The control group received no specific intervention. <u>Outcome Measures</u> ▪ Pittsburgh Agitation Scale ▪ Spatial orientation subscale ▪ Study-designed outcome, to measure residents' ability to find way to the dining room and bedroom	More residents in the intervention group were able to find their way to the dining room compared with those in the control group ($p = .03$) 1 wk after intervention, but this was not sustained at 3 mo after intervention. There were no differences between groups in finding their way to their bedrooms. Both groups had significantly decreased agitation at posttest 1 ($p = .04$), suggesting that both groups benefited from the relocation in terms of their agitation. At 3 mo after intervention, residents in the treatment group had significantly higher agitation than those in the control group ($p = .024$). Spatial orientation scores were low for both groups. The control group's scores declined over time more than the intervention group, but the difference was not statistically significant.	The authors identify that a larger sample size would be beneficial. There is possible attention bias because the intervention group received more attention than the control group. In addition, the site of the intervention may also bias results because different residents may live different distances from the dining room and this distance may influence whether the resident learned or not (i.e., more complex route may have decreased residents' ability to find their way).	The results of this study support the potential short-term efficacy of a way-finding program on the residents' ability to locate an intended destination and the need for ongoing intervention. The use of location maps was anecdotally reported to be less useful in assisting with way finding, but further exploration of this is warranted. This study suggests that this type of program could be carried out by paraprofessional staff with the supervision of professional staff, and similarly this protocol could be taught to families, which would be particularly beneficial if there were a language barrier, and since it appears that regular intervention may be needed to sustain the way-finding successes.

McGilton, K. S., Rivera, T. M., & Dawson, P. (2003). Can we help persons with dementia find their way in a new environment? *Aging and Mental Health, 7,* 363–371.

| Namazi & Johnson, 1992a | The aim of the study was to generate evidence that visual barriers in the environment are beneficial for individuals with AD. | Level III
Quasi experimental, 1-group randomized crossover design

Participants
12 residents of the Corinne Dolan Alzheimer Center were enrolled in the study. | Intervention
3 barrier heights were randomly assigned. Each participant participated in 12 trials. 2 participants were tested in each 20-min trial period.

Participants were grouped into categories on the basis of MMSE score. A trained observer observed participants for 4 trials of each condition, 20 min at a time for 4 wk.

Group 1: 78-in. removable divider

Group 2: 54-in. removable divider

Group 3: No barrier

For all participants, age-appropriate color-by-number art projects were selected for 11 of the 12 participants. The 12th participant was not able to engage in the art project, and coin sorting was a substituted activity for this person.

Outcome Measures
The authors describe 7 categories of distractions that were tallied by the observer if the participant engaged in them for > 5 s. | There was a reduction in the overall number of auditory distractions in the low and high barrier conditions. The high barrier reduced distractions more than the low barrier.

Participants with lower MMSE scores were more distracted than the other groups. | There were biases in sample selection because participants were encouraged to participate in the study.

Psychometric properties of the outcome measure are not reported.

The authors were not able to explain the anomaly in the data, which showed that the low barrier may have adversely affected attention in the group of participants with the lowest MMSE scores.

Further research is required to replicate these findings with a higher level of evidence. | An interesting implication for occupational therapy arising from this study is the ability of people with moderate to mild AD to attend to a task that is meaningful and dignified (an average of 16 out of 20 min). This attention was enhanced in most cases by the use of a visual barrier, which also decreased attending to auditory distractions. This has implications for possible use in residences where there are often large common areas used for group programming, and also possibly for home use in helping a person stay on task with dressing, eating, or other ADLs/IADLs. In addition, it could be used in a busy household to decrease attention to irrelevant auditory stimuli. The barriers have the benefit of being relatively inexpensive and portable. |

Namazi, K. H., & Johnson, B. D. (1992a). The effects of environmental barriers on the attention span of Alzheimer's disease patients. *American Journal of Alzheimer's Care and Related Disorders and Research, 7,* 9–15.

(continued)

EVIDENCE TABLE: What is the evidence for the effect of interventions designed to modify and maintain perceptual abilities on the occupational performance of people with dementia? *(continued)*

Author/Year	Study Objectives	Level/Design/ Participants	Intervention and Outcome Measures	Results	Study Limitations	Implications for Occupational Therapy
Namazi & Johnson, 1992b	The purpose of the study was to identify features of the environment, which can support the remaining abilities of persons with AD, and to address the issue of decision making and pertinent autonomy. Specifically, the study measured changes in residents' behaviors when they encountered both locked and unlocked exit doors.	Level III 1 group, comparing responses of 2 door set-ups Participants Participants were 22 residents of a long-term-care facility with dementia. Inclusion/ exclusion criteria not provided.	Intervention The intervention was an unlocked exit door to an outside courtyard. The control condition was the locked door. Each condition was present for 50 hr of observation; 3 hr in the morning and 3 hr in the afternoon. Outcome Measures A study-designed observational checklist was use to observe participant responses to the 2 door conditions. 5 categories of behaviors were observed.	Results report on the first 30 min after residents encountered the locked or unlocked door. Under the locked door condition, there were 1,417 active responses and 114 verbal responses. Under the unlocked door conditions, there were 393 active responses and 25 verbal responses. Differences between the 2 conditions were not tested for statistical significance.	Limited information was provided about the study sample and the measures used. Observation of behaviors does not seem to be compatible with the study purpose of supporting remaining abilities, or addressing the issue of decision making and autonomy. Limited information was provided on participant recruitment or inclusion/exclusion criteria. The sample size was not justified. The duration of the study was not clearly described. The results are descriptive only—very little can be concluded about the value of an unlocked door in changing behaviors.	The results of this study suggest that an unlocked exit door may reduce unwanted behaviors in residents with Alzheimer's disease and other dementias. Because no statistical significance was reported, this conclusion must be interpreted with caution. The authors' conclusions related to autonomy, decision making, and quality of life seem inappropriate considering the study and measurement limitations. The study provides limited support for the notion that environmental design can influence behaviors or occupational performance (e.g., walking, verbal communication). The study does not provide a link between the environmental condition and using remaining perceptual abilities.

Namazi, K. H., & Johnson, B. D. (1992b). Pertinent autonomy for residents with dementias: Modification of the physical environment to enhance independence. *American Journal of Alzheimer's Care and Related Disorders and Research, 7,* 16–21.

| Namazi, Rosner, & Calkins, 1989 | The objective was to examine whether visual barriers would stop residents with AD from leaving the unit through an emergency door. | <u>Level III</u>
Before-and-after design (nonrandomized)

<u>Participants</u>
A convenience sample of 9 residents in a 30-bed unit with a diagnosis of dementia and symptoms of visual agnosia on neurological examination | <u>Intervention</u>
Baseline data on exit behavior were collected 2 wk before study with no barriers at exit door and fire exit door had a turn knob. For 14 days, participants were exposed to various barriers, including visual barriers based on optical illusion using strips of black, beige, or brown tape; barriers involving concealment of the knob or a doorknob cover that requires applied pressure to open it was placed over the doorknob. Participants were not exposed to any visual barriers to examine potential learning effects of prior barriers.

<u>Outcome Measures</u>
A record of the number of times a resident attempted to open and exit the door. | Less exiting occurred when the barriers involving concealment of the knob were used (i.e. the cloth barriers, both beige and green patterned, were associated with no exits and the beige painted knob was associated with 14 exits and the knob cover with 7).

When participants were exposed to a replication of baseline conditions (i.e., no barrier), there was a decrease in exits to 22 from a reported 43 at baseline. | The sample size in the study was not justified by a power analysis.

Results were reported in terms of descriptive data, and the study sample was small and homogenous.

The authors also pointed out that the clinician should examine individual characteristics to best develop management techniques. Hence, this technique may not generalize but could be successful with residents sharing the characteristics of participants in this study. | The results of this study imply that full concealment of an exit doorknob with cloth, irrespective of contrast, may reduce or eliminate exiting for persons with severe dementia (as measured by MMSE) and symptoms of visual agnosia. It was only tested on a residential unit, but strategies may also work in private homes.

In terms of cost-effectiveness and delivery, these types of methods are appealing. They support the independence and dignity of residents with dementia, while optimizing safety and possible decreasing the work of staff. |

Namazi, K. H., Rosner, T. T., & Calkins, M. P. (1989). Visual barriers to prevent ambulatory Alzheimer's patients from exiting through an emergency door. *Gerontologist, 29*(5), 699–702.

(continued)

EVIDENCE TABLE: What is the evidence for the effect of interventions designed to modify and maintain perceptual abilities on the occupational performance of people with dementia? *(continued)*

Author/Year	Study Objectives	Level/Design/ Participants	Intervention and Outcome Measures	Results	Study Limitations	Implications for Occupational Therapy
Pankow, Pliskin, & Luchins, 1996	The objective was to report the possible benefit of optical intervention for treatment of visual hallucinations in older adults with the combined diagnoses of visual impairment and dementia.	<u>Level IV</u> Case series design <u>Participants</u> *Inclusion Criteria:* Purposeful selection of 3 participants who had been referred for low-vision evaluations by the psychiatry and neuropsychology services. Each patient had an ocular pathology after eye exam and a dementia diagnosis supported by neuropsychology tests.	<u>Intervention</u> Trial of visual aids, including (a) telescopic devices, handheld or spectacle mounted, to improve distance vision; (b) high-powered plus lenses to improve near vision; (c) tints and lighting changes to reduce photophobia and enhanced contrast; (d) spectacle-mounted prisms to expand limited peripheral vision. The intervention was provided once. The duration of the intervention was 15 wk for Case 1 and 3 and 9 wk for Case 2. In addition, there was a trial of nonoptical aids (bold-lined paper, large-print materials, and check stencils) for meeting patient goals related to vision. <u>Outcome Measures</u> The Hallucination questionnaire	<u>Case 1:</u> Baseline—hallucinations reported 1×/hr. After receiving the optical aid, the hallucinations decreased to 1–3× / day over the 13 wk of follow-up. The patient reported being less upset by the remaining hallucinations. <u>Case 2:</u> Baseline hallucinations reported at 1×/hr. After receiving his optical aid, the hallucinations decreased to 1–3×/day. Also, he reported being less upset. <u>Case 3:</u> Baseline—hallucinations reported at 2×/day. After receiving instruction on use of visual aids, the hallucinations decreased in the range of 2–3×/wk to 1×/day.	There is a potential for referral bias and Hawthorne effect because participants were all referred to participate in the study. The only outcome measure used was a self-report questionnaire. This leads to a possible bias, because all participants and family were aware that these interventions were aimed at decreasing hallucinations.	This study, although preliminary, suggests that for clients with dementia and a visual impairment, optical and visual aids may be helpful in reducing hallucinations and improving daily functioning. Some interventions may require an optical specialist. Environmental changes can be implemented by occupational therapists, although these were not discussed in the case studies.

Pankow, L., Pliskin, N., & Luchins, D. (1996). An optical intervention for visual hallucinations associated with visual impairments and dementia in elderly patients. *Journal of Neuropsychiatry, 8,* 88–92.

Passini, Pigot, Rainville, & Tetreault, 2000	The objectives of the study were ■ To identify residual way-finding abilities in people with advanced DAT To identify architectural, interior design, and graphic features that cause way-finding difficulties or that facilitate mobility in people with DAT ■ To identify aspects of nursing home care that impinge on spatial mobility of patients with DAT	Level IV Multiple case study with residents; 1-time interviews with staff Participants 6 residents of a nursing home who satisfied the inclusion criteria were selected by staff for the study.	Intervention The intervention was the nursing home environment. Each resident participant was to go to a specific destination that was identified on a memory aid (4 tasks that ranged in complexity and familiarity). Participants were instructed not to ask other people for information. An observer walked with the participant and ensured the participant verbalized his or her thought and decision-making process. A second observer followed and noted on a floor plan behavioral particularities. The conversation between the first observer and the participant was also recorded. 10 staff members from various disciplines were interviewed based on a questionnaire in a semi-structured manner. Outcome Measures A study-designed outcome measure was used.	Staff members' perception is that current signage does not necessarily address the needs of the patient because of size, location, and complexity of the information. Way-finding data suggest that signs may help provide directional information to remind patients where facilities are located and how to return to their points of origin and that the use of pictograms warrants further research. Finally, it is important that the name of a place be consistent, relate to its function, and reflect the cultural particularities of the patients as much as possible. Reactions to floor surfaces are individual; however, the research suggests the avoidance of dark patterns as well as any decisive separation of 1 area from the other. Designs that encourage way finding only make sense if the patients are encouraged to use the setting as intended.	The authors did not state how the sample was recruited, so selection bias is possible. The staff members working in the nursing home helped select the residents for the study. This may have influenced the results, because there is potential to select residents who would either do very well or do poorly. The study did not describe whether the same person acted as the observer or whether different people took on this role. Inadequate information was provided on psychometric properties of the measures. Limited sample and low level of evidence make generalization of results difficult.	This study provided numerous suggestions to create a supportive way-finding environment for patients with advanced AD. However, the authors drew many conclusions and recommendations for design changes that were not substantiated in their paper, and the results should be interpreted with caution.

Passini, R., Pigot, H., Rainville, C., & Tetreault, M. (2000). Way finding in a nursing home for advanced dementia of the Alzheimer's type. *Environment and Behavior, 32*, 684–710.

(continued)

EVIDENCE TABLE: What is the evidence for the effect of interventions designed to modify and maintain perceptual abilities on the occupational performance of people with dementia? *(continued)*

Author/Year	Study Objectives	Level/Design/ Participants	Intervention and Outcome Measures	Results	Study Limitations	Implications for Occupational Therapy
Passini, Rainville, Marchand, & Joanette, 1998	The objective was to identify way-finding abilities of patients with DAT at the early and middle stages of dementia in respect to decision making and information processing.	Level II Cohort study Participants 14 participants in the intervention group, 28 in the control group Intervention group participants were people with DAT. Control group members were matched older adults with no cognitive impairment.	Intervention At a geriatric institute (Hospital Cote-des-Neiges), participants had to start from the closest bus stop in front of the hospital and find their way to the hospital dental clinic. After reaching the clinic, they were to return to the bus stop using the same route. An observer accompanied each participant. The participants were asked to verbalize everything that went through their mind while reaching the destination. Conversations were recorded and transcribed. Outcome Measures Specific measure were not described. The study refers to using a "Typology of Decision Based on Environmental Information (Type A) and Typology of Exploratory Decisions (Type B)" to analyze the type of decision making participants used.	Trip to clinic: 12 of 14 participants experimental participants needed > 3 interventions. 21 of 28 control participants needed no intervention. Return trip to bus stop: Experimental group: No change Control group: 24 of 28 participants needed no intervention. Decision type analysis: Decisions based on memory were noted to be present more in the control group. Looking and walking without aim was only present for the experimental group. Exploring to find the destination directly was more by the experimental group. Exploring to find specific information was done by both groups, but more by the control group. Return trip: There was a large shift from exploratory to memory-based decisions for the control group. 88.45% of all control group decisions were decisions based on memory, whereas the DAT group had a similar distribution to the first half of the trip.	Limited information regarding data collection and analyses make it difficult to determine whether the study was adequately powered. Not stated if the observer was 1 or more people. Generalizability of the results is limited, given the limited information provided on sample characteristics, possible biases, and limitations to the study design.	Considering limitations related to measurement and analyses, major redesigns of buildings can not be justified based on this study. This study suggests that appropriately designed environments may improve way finding and quality of life for persons with dementia. It can be hypothesized that appropriately designed environments may delay admissions to nursing homes and possibly allow nursing homes to be more cost effective. Further research necessary to explore how the recommendations made by the authors enhance way-finding abilities in persons with dementia.

Passini, R., Rainville, C., Marchand, N., & Joanette, Y. (1998). Way finding and dementia: Some research findings and a new look at design. *Journal of Architectural and Planning Research, 15*, 133–151.

Summary of Quantitative Evidence: Routines

EVIDENCE TABLE: What is the evidence for the effectiveness of interventions designed to establish, modify, or maintain routines on the occupational performance, quality of life, health and wellness, and client and caregiver satisfaction of persons with Alzheimer's disease?

Author/Year	Study Objectives	Level/Design/ Participants	Intervention and Outcome Measures	Results	Study Limitations	Implications for Occupational Therapy
Evidence on routines in general						
Kovach & Stearns, 1994	The objective was to determine whether there was a difference in behaviors associated with dementia before and after move to a dementia SCU and to determine whether the need for chemical or physical restraint was different after move to an SCU.	<u>Level III</u> Before-and-after design <u>Participants</u> 24 residents scheduled to move to a new unit were recruited. Admission criteria for the unit were as follows: resident with mild to severe irreversible cognitive impairment; resident who exhibits anxiety, agitation, affective disturbances or activity disturbances when in an unstructured environment; resident who experiences social isolation or diversional activity deficit when not engaged in group programs; resident who can engage in group programming or not be disruptive to group activities	<u>Intervention</u> SCU involved specialized activities to meet individual treatment goals and a planned schedule of activities; activities to promote maximum functioning; a safe environment adapted to the needs of the residents. Intervention offered by a multidisciplinary team. <u>Outcome Measures</u> ■ Behavioral Pathology in Alzheimer's Disease Rating Scale BEHAVE-AD (modified) ■ Restraint record	Significant reduction was reported in activity disturbances, aggression, affective disturbances, and increase in social interactions on the modified BEHAVE-AD—mean of 8.0 at pretest and 4 at posttest (paired t test: $p < .001$). In a global ranking of how troubling or dangerous behavior was, 9 patients ranked as mild before and 2 after, and 1 was moderate before and 2 were moderate after. 4 patients increased their use of physical restraints, whereas 5 became restraint free and 6 required the same level of physical restraints. No participants decreased their use of chemical restraints; 2 increased dosages and 4 remained the same. 5 patients increased phobic behavior, but no value was reported.	Single-group design makes it impossible to compare the effect of the CSU to other factors. Other, similar clients may have experienced similar changes in outcomes without being moved to a SCU. The multimodal intervention makes it impossible to identify whether the routine offered on the CSU was a major contributor to the changes notes. The occupational therapy role on the unit was not clearly outlined, and occupational therapy is not listed as a discipline with a lead role in implementing the activities routine on the unit. Modifications to the BEHAVE-AD were not well described; information about reliability and validity was not provided.	Although routines are only 1 aspect of the SCU, this study provides some support (although preliminary) for the value of the SCU in reducing some challenging behaviors and the use of physical restraints. The study did not examine outcomes related to occupational performance, quality of life, health and wellness, and client and caregiver satisfaction.

Kovach, C. R., & Stearns, S. A. (1994). DSCUS: A study of behavior before and after residence. *Journal of Gerontological Nursing, 29*, 33–39.

(continued)

Summary of Quantitative Evidence: Routines

EVIDENCE TABLE: What is the evidence for the effectiveness of interventions designed to establish, modify, or maintain routines on the occupational performance, quality of life, health and wellness, and client and caregiver satisfaction of persons with Alzheimer's disease? *(continued)*

Author/Year	Study Objectives	Level/Design/ Participants	Intervention and Outcome Measures	Results	Study Limitations	Implications for Occupational Therapy
Evidence on toileting routines						
Doody, Stevens, Beck, Dubinsky, Kaye, Gwyther, et al., 2001	The objective was to review the evidence and provide recommendations for the management of dementia, including pharmacological and nonpharmacological interventions. Relevant to the focused question, the review asked, "Do nonpharmacological interventions, other than education, improve outcomes in patients or caregivers of patients with dementia compared with no such interventions?"	Level I Evidence-based review	Intervention Review included behavior modification, prompted voiding, and scheduled toileting.	2 studies demonstrated that behavior modification, scheduled toileting, and prompted voiding can reduce urinary incontinence. The review panel members felt that the evidence was strong enough that they recommended the use of these strategies as standard practice.	The link of reduced incontinence to quality of life, occupational performance, or satisfaction was not discussed. 1 study cited as a primary data source is a review (Skelly & Flint, 1995), and the second is a book chapter that may not be a study report.	Occupational therapists and occupational therapy assistants, when working with people with dementia, need to be alert to any toileting routines being implemented to ensure adherence. Clients or caregivers with problems related to toileting may want to consider implementing such routines (at least on a pilot basis) to reduce incontinence. However, evidence from this review is not strong, considering the limitations.

Doody, R. S., Stevens, J. C., Beck, C., Dubinsky, R. M., Kaye, J. A., Gwyther, L., et al. (2001). Practice parameter: Management of dementia (an evidence-based review). Report of the Quality Standards Subcommittee of the American Academy of Neurology. *Neurology, 56,* 1154–1166.

| Eustice, Roe, & Paterson, 2000 | The objective was to determine the effectiveness and efficiency of prompted voiding for the management of urinary incontinence. | Level I Systematic review (Cochrane) Included all randomized or quasi-randomized trials of prompted voiding for the management of urinary incontinence. | Intervention Prompted voiding involved a routine of asking the resident about the need to use the toilet, and providing assistance to the resident to do so. | 6 studies were included in the review; however, no results were provided in 1. The sample described included 355 older adults (296 or 83% women), with an average age of 82 yr. The studies provided no evidence for long-term effects of the interventions. Data were extracted from 3 trials involving a total of 82 participants in the treatment group and 84 in the control group favored prompted voiding compared with no prompted voiding, although the difference was not statistically significant. 1 trial reported a statistically significant increase in independent requests for the toilet as a result of the prompted voiding intervention. | The link of reduced incontinence to quality of life, occupational performance, or satisfaction was not discussed in any of the studies included in this systematic review. | This systematic review suggested that prompted voiding may be helpful in reducing incontinence. Occupational therapists and occupational therapy assistants working in these settings and occupational therapy students need to be familiar with the principles of prompted voiding, so that their interventions are planned in order to enable its use. Further, occupational therapists should consider interventions directed toward environmental modifications to promote mobility and safe toilet use in settings implementing prompted voiding. |

Eustice, S., Roe, B., & Paterson, J. (2000). Prompted voiding for the management of urinary incontinence in adults. *Cochrane Database of Systematic Reviews*, Issue 2. Art. No.: CD002113. doi: 10.1002/14651858.CD002113

(continued)

Summary of Quantitative Evidence: Routines

EVIDENCE TABLE: What is the evidence for the effectiveness of interventions designed to establish, modify, or maintain routines on the occupational performance, quality of life, health and wellness, and client and caregiver satisfaction of persons with Alzheimer's disease? *(continued)*

Author/Year	Study Objectives	Level/Design/ Participants	Intervention and Outcome Measures	Results	Study Limitations	Implications for Occupational Therapy
Ostaszkiewicz, Johnston, & Roe, 2004a	The objective was to assess the effectiveness of habit retraining for the management of urinary incontinence in adults.	Level I Systematic Review (Cochrane) Included all randomized or quasi-randomized trials of habit retraining for the management of urinary incontinence in adults.	Intervention Habit retraining is a form of maintaining the habits or routines related to voiding for people with dementia. It is individualized based on the routines of each person.	Total of 3 studies (RCTs–Level I) were included in the review. The sample described included 1 study with 113 older adults in a long-term-care facility, and 2 studies with 224 home-based community-dwelling older adults. Across the 3 studies, the average age was 80.3 yr, and primarily included women with cognitive or physical impairments who were dependent on caregivers. Of the 3 trials reviewed, data from 1 study could not be completely analyzed because of reporting methods. Data from a second study showed nonsignificant between-group differences in incontinent episodes, whereas data from the third study favored the intervention group with no statistically significant differences between the groups. 1 trial evaluated caregiver burden and noted that caregivers reported the management of incontinence to be less stressful at the end of the intervention than at baseline, although there were no significant changes during the trial period.	All 3 studies included in the review reported problems with adherence to treatment protocols and data collection tools. The quality of the trials was modest with poor reporting on levels of concealment to allocation, interventions, and outcome assessment as each trial had missing data, high attrition, and analyses based on complete cases rather than ITT analyses.	Although habit retraining fits very well with occupational therapy as a client-centered strategy to maintain routines for people with dementia, this systematic review did not find strong evidence to support or refute its adoption. It seems that the implementation of habit retraining requires commitment and resources by caregivers (formal or informal) to implement.

Ostaszkiewicz, J., Johnston, L., & Roe, B. (2004a). Habit retraining for the management of urinary incontinence in adults. *Cochrane Database of Systematic Reviews*, Issue 2. Art. No.: CD002801.pub2. doi: 10.1002/14651858.CD002801.pub2

Reference	Objective	Level/Design	Intervention	Findings	
Ostaszkiewicz, Johnston, & Roe, 2004b	The objective was to assess the effectiveness of timed voiding for the management of urinary incontinence in adults.	Level I Systematic review (Cochrane) or quasi-randomized trials of timed voiding for the management of urinary incontinence.	Intervention Timed voiding is thought to be most useful for people who are not able to participate in toileting or who cannot communicate the need to void. It involves regularly toileting the person to avoid incontinent events. It is typically used in long-term-care facilities.	2 trials were included: most participants in both selected trials were older women (mean age 86.7) with cognitive impairment. All resided in nursing facilities. In 1 trial, fewer incontinence events were noted in the intervention group, but between-group comparisons were not completed. There were significantly fewer wet-checks noted in the intervention compared to the control group, but no standard deviation was reported. In the second trial, with a larger sample size, between-group differences were statistically significant for nighttime incontinence but not for daytime.	Methodological quality of these trials was not high, particularly related to a lack of clarity regarding levels of blinding.
					The review found little evidence to support or refute the use of timed voiding. Although it may be useful in circumstances of working with people who are not able to identify or communicate their need to void, its adoption needs to be considered in terms of the ability to adhere to a regular schedule and how residents respond to such routines.

Ostaszkiewicz, J., Johnston, L., & Roe, B. (2004b). Timed voiding for the management of urinary incontinence in adults. *Cochrane Database of Systematic Reviews*, Issue 1. Art. No.: CD002802.pub2. DOI: 10.1002/14651858.CD002802.pub2

(continued)

Summary of Quantitative Evidence: Routines

EVIDENCE TABLE: What is the evidence for the effectiveness of interventions designed to establish, modify, or maintain routines on the occupational performance, quality of life, health and wellness, and client and caregiver satisfaction of persons with Alzheimer's disease? *(continued)*

Author/Year	Study Objectives	Level/Design/ Participants	Intervention and Outcome Measures	Results	Study Limitations	Implications for Occupational Therapy
Skelly, J., & Flint, 1995	The objective was to critically review literature on urinary incontinence associated with AD and vascular (multi-infarct) dementia, with particular reference to its prevalence, etiology, assessment, and management.	Level V Narrative review Inclusion and exclusion criteria for studies reviewed not clearly stated.	Intervention The review included studies of 3 types of toileting routines (scheduled toileting, habit retraining, prompted voided).	1 uncontrolled trial found a 26% decrease in episodes of incontinence in its participants with the use of fixed scheduled toileting. 1 controlled trial found a 19% decrease in episodes of incontinence; 2 uncontrolled trials (pre–post studies) found, respectively, a 55% decrease in episodes of incontinence in its participants, whereas the second found no change in its participants with the use of individualized scheduled toileting. In 3 RCTs of prompted voiding, incontinence decreased from 26–50% for people in the experimental groups in nursing homes. Similar decreases were noted in other less rigorous evaluations of prompted voiding.	This review is based on studies published from 1970–1994. Limited information is provided about the literature search strategies used. Clear inclusion and exclusion criteria for studies included in the review were not reported. No information was provided about the methods of data extraction or quality assessment of the studies included. Outcomes focus on continence, but no link was made between toileting routines and quality of life, health and well-being, and client or caregiver satisfaction.	The authors concluded that prompted voiding regimens reduce incontinence by an average of 32% and appear to be useful to managing incontinence in some patients with dementia. The conclusions about the effectiveness of prompted voiding seem to be valid for residents of nursing homes. For occupational therapists in clinical practice, it is important to be aware of any routines related to toileting, such as prompted voiding, so that adherence to the schedule is maintained.

Skelly, J., & Flint, A. J. (1995). Urinary incontinence associated with dementia. *Journal of the American Geriatrics Society, 43*, 286–294.

Evidence on sleep routines

Author/Year	Study Objectives	Level/Design/ Participants	Intervention and Outcome Measures	Results	Study Limitations	Implications for Occupational Therapy
Alessi, Martin, Webber, Kim, Harker, & Josephson, 2005	The objective was to test a multidimensional, nonpharmacological intervention to improve sleep–wake patterns, and indirectly quality of life, by targeting multiple contributing factors in sleep disruption and to design an intervention that would be feasible to implement in a nursing home (clinical applicability).	Level I RCT Participants *n* = 118 ≥ 15% observed daytime sleep over 2 days ≤ 80% nighttime sleep over 2 nights (using wrist actigraphy) Criteria were based on normative data in healthy people.	Intervention The intervention group encouraged patients to remain out of bed during the day; daily exposure to sunlight ≥ 10,000 lux; participation in low-level physical activity program; installation of a bedtime routine; reduced nighttime noise and light in hallways and sleeping rooms; and decreased personal care through the night by nursing. Outcome Measures ■ Actillume wrist actigraphy ■ Structured behavioral observation ■ Bedside monitor	No statistically significant differences between intervention and control groups in nighttime total sleep, percentage of sleep, or number of awakenings was reported. A decrease in mean awakening length (min) in the intervention group was significant at $p = .04$. A decrease (46%) in observed daytime sleeping was significant at $p < .001$, and no change was observed in controls. Percentage of observed participation in social activities was significantly greater in the intervention group ($p < .001$) and the percentage of observed participation in physical activities was also significantly increased in the intervention group ($p = .001$). There was a trend for increased participation in social conversation in the intervention group. No significant differences were noted for agitation or level of assistance required when eating or drinking.	Diagnoses were not described, except to say that the sample was typical of nursing home residents, with cognitive impairment and co-morbidities. Members of the control group did not receive an attention control. The authors note that this might have contributed to their circadian rhythms and inadvertently been a form of contamination.	Although a multimodal intervention for sleep disturbance may prove most effective, it is unfortunate that bedtime routine was not examined alone for its impact. As such, this intervention must be taken as a whole. However, changing one's living pattern to include exposure to light, increase physical activity, limit in-bed time during the day, and establish a personalized bedtime routine could all be considered to be aspects of a larger daily routine. Occupational therapists working in nursing home settings may be able to work with the nursing team to develop strategies and education to implement this type of multimodal approach. This study suggests that the intervention may contribute to indicators of quality of life, even if the amount of nighttime sleep is not altered. However, the long-term effects of the intervention have not been examined, nor have implementation costs been considered.

Alessi, C. A., Martin, J. L., Webber, A. P., Kim, E. C., Harker, J. O., & Josephson, K. R. (2005). Randomized, controlled trial of a non-pharmacological intervention to improve abnormal sleep/ wake patterns in nursing home residents. *Journal of the American Geriatrics Society, 53*, 803–810.

(continued)

Summary of Quantitative Evidence: Routines

EVIDENCE TABLE: What is the evidence for the effectiveness of interventions designed to establish, modify, or maintain routines on the occupational performance, quality of life, health and wellness, and client and caregiver satisfaction of persons with Alzheimer's disease? *(continued)*

Author/Year	Study Objectives	Level/Design/ Participants	Intervention and Outcome Measures	Results	Study Limitations	Implications for Occupational Therapy
McCurry, Gibbons, Logsdon, Vitiello, & Teri, 2003	The objective was to determine whether caregivers can be trained to use sleep hygiene (e.g., reducing daytime sleep and improving the sleep environment and nighttime routine) recommendations in patients with dementia residing in the community.	Level I RCT Participants *n* = 22 All participants met the NINCDS–ADRDA criteria for probable or possible Alzheimer's disease confirmed in writing by their primary care physicians. They were living at home with a family caregiver.	Intervention 10 patients and their caregivers were given 6 in-home sessions with a geropsychologist over 2 mo, including written materials and individualized program of sleep hygiene techniques. Specific sleep hygiene recommendations were negotiated with the caregiver, and follow-up sessions involved problem-solving with the caregiver to implement the sleep hygiene recommendations. Outcome Measures Daily sleep logs to measure sleep hygiene adherence.	Consistency of bedtime was achieved in 83% of intervention vs. 38% of control participants (*p* = .0024); rising time consistency was 96% vs. 59% (*p* = .0092); reduction of patient napping 70% vs. 28% (*p* = .0066); institution of walking program 86% vs. 7% (*p* < .0001).	Because the analyses are based on "target" participants only (i.e., those deemed to need to make changes in sleep routines), it is difficult to know the differences between all members of the 2 groups. Information about the effects of the intervention is not provided in this study.	Occupational therapists working in home-care environments with clients with dementia and their caregivers should inquire about routines related to sleep as part of the assessment process, and support caregivers to set and address goals in this area of daily routine as required.

McCurry, S. M., Gibbons, L. E., Logsdon, R. G., Vitiello, M., & Teri, L. (2003). Training caregivers to change the sleep hygiene practices of patients with dementia: The NITE–AD project. *Journal of the American Geriatrics Society, 51,* 1455–1460.

		Intervention	Outcome	
McCurry, Gibbons, Logsdon, Vitiello, & Teri, 2005	The objective was to evaluate whether a comprehensive sleep education program (NITE-AD) could improve sleep in dementia patients living at home with their family caregivers.	Level I RCT Participants $n = 36$ All participants met the NINCDS-ADRDA criteria for probable or possible Alzheimer's disease confirmed in writing by their primary care physicians.	Intervention Intervention included sleep hygiene education, goal setting, and intervention related to sleep hygiene (setting a regular sleep routine, avoiding daytime sleeping); daily walking and light exposure (using a light box) over 3 weekly sessions; followed by monitoring and assistance for biweekly sessions over the following 6 wk. Outcome Measures ■ Actillume wrist-movement recorder ■ Pittsburgh Sleep Quality Index ■ Epworth Sleepiness Scale ■ Cornell Depression Scale ■ CES-D ■ RMBPC	At 2 mo and 6 mo, statistically significant differences favoring the intervention group were noted for nighttime waking with less awake time ($p = .03$), fewer night awakenings ($p = .01$), fewer wakes/hr ($p = .03$), and smaller duration of night awakenings ($p = .04$). Caregivers in the intervention group reported significantly more daily exercise ($p = .01$), more caregiver exercise ($p = .07$), and significantly lower depression ratings on the RMBPC ($p = .007$).	Power calculations not reported in the study. Although results are statistically significant (suggesting adequate power because differences between groups were significant), the sample size seems small for the number of outcomes measured.	It appears that the intervention was effective in improving nighttime sleep and is worthwhile considering as part of an intervention related to daily routines for people with dementia. The intervention included sleep routines, daily walking, and light therapy, so the relative contribution of each of these components cannot be determined on the basis of these results. The training provided to caregivers was brief, and with follow-up it was maintained, suggesting that it is feasible to offer in a community setting.

McCurry, S. M., Gibbons, L. E., Logsdon, R. G., Vitiello, M. V., & Teri, L. (2005). Nighttime insomnia treatment and education for Alzheimer's disease: A randomized controlled trial. *Journal of the American Geriatrics Society, 53*, 793–802.

(continued)

Qualitative Evidence: Routines

EVIDENCE TABLE: What is the evidence for the effectiveness of interventions designed to establish, modify, or maintain routines on the occupational performance, quality of life, health and wellness, and client and caregiver satisfaction of persons with Alzheimer's disease?

Author/Year	Study Objectives	Design and Participants	Findings	Trustworthiness/ Limitations	Implications for Occupational Therapy
Donovan & Dupuis, 2000	The purpose of the study was to explore perceptions of family and staff about why a SCU had resulted in positive change for residents, which had been documented in a pre–post evaluation of the unit. (Note the positive changes are never specifically described.)	Qualitative interviews were conducted with 8 staff members and 17 family members of residents of a 24-bed SCU for people with dementia in New Brunswick, Canada.	3 major reasons for the SCU's positive influence on residents' behaviors were noted: (1) feelings of having a personal space designated for each resident for personal use and private socializing; (2) expressions of personhood were fostered by having staff familiar with the life story of each resident and being well-trained regarding dementia; and (3) unforced routines, which were characterized by residents' choosing their own schedules, staff not assigned to provide care to specific residents, equipping the unit with a kitchen to enable reheating of meals or simple snack preparation, and support from administration and family members.	There is limited information provided about how participants in the study were recruited, and little information about their characteristics is provided. Data collection and analyses are described very briefly, with little information related to rigor or credibility reported. Findings that are shared are primarily descriptive with little interpretation.	The findings are not strong enough to make recommendations for clinical implementation. Philosophically, unforced routines fit very nicely with ideas underlying client-centered (rather than staff-centered) care. Further rigorous research is needed to investigate the transferability of these findings to other settings.

Donovan, C., & Dupuis, M. (2000). Specialized care unit: Family and staff perceptions of significant elements. *Geriatric Nursing, 21,* 30–33.

Author/Year	Study Objectives	Design and Participants	Findings	Trustworthiness/ Limitations	Implications for Occupational Therapy
Gotell, Brown, & Ekman, 2002	The study examined whether or not the use of background music or singing by a caregiver enhanced understanding of and cooperation with the morning care routine.	Phenomenological study involving video recording of morning care routines under 3 conditions: usual care, background music, and caregiver singing. Participants included 9 residents of a SCU in Sweden and 5 staff providing their care.	Verbal interactions were reduced in both music-based situations (both when background music was played and when the caregiver was singing or humming). However, in both music-based situations, residents seemed to require less cueing (verbal or nonverbal) to understand and participate more actively and willingly in the morning care routines.	Because only 4 of 9 dyads were presented, it is unclear whether these were the only interactions that illustrated the differences between the 3 situations. Inadequate information was provided about the data collection methods and analyses.	Music programming during daily routines may be a valuable addition in long-term-care settings for people with severe dementia, but program evaluation is warranted. The use of music may have changed the milieu of the interaction and it is the different milieu to which the participants responded (e.g., caregivers engaging in singing or humming can not simultaneously talk to others).

Gotell, E., Brown, S., & Ekman, S. L. (2002). Caregiver singing and background music in dementia care. *Western Journal of Nursing Research, 24,* 195–216.

Hutchinson, Leger-Krall, & Wilson, 1996	The study aimed to answer the following questions: ■ What is the range and variation of toileting problems? ■ What management strategies are used by family and employed caregivers? ■ What interactive and contextual conditions influence the experience and management strategies?	The study was described as an ethnology undertaken in a day care center for people with AD, located in a large southeastern U.S. city. An average daily census of 21 clients participated at the center. The staff to patient ratio was 1:5. Participant observations were conducted in the center with an unspecified number of clients. Interviews were conducted with 13 staff and 16 family members.	This study provided a rich description of the experiences of clients, staff, and to a lesser extent, family members, in relation to toileting experiences. Use of toileting routines designed to meet individual client needs can reduce the incidence of toileting problems.	Many details related to the methods of data collection and analyses were not reported, and study limitations and author biases/assumptions were not explicitly discussed by the authors. The limitations in the description of the methods and analyses make it difficult to feel confident about the conclusions of the authors.	Suggestions for practice in a day care center include the following: ■ Follow routine toileting ■ Be alert to verbal and behavioral cues ■ Respond to cues from clients ■ Regularly communicate with families

Hutchinson, S., Leger-Krall, S., & Wilson, H. S. (1996). Toileting: A biobehavioral challenge in Alzheimer's dementia care. *Journal of Gerontological Nursing, 22*, 18–27.

Nygård & Johansson, 2001	The objective was to describe the experience and management of time and temporal problems in everyday life of a small group of individuals with dementia and to describe the process and results of interventions using time aids (e.g., adaptive clocks, medicine dosettes, and special calendars).	Phenomenological study involving 5 people with dementia seen as outpatients. Interviews were conducted at baseline and after provision of intervention to address temporal problems.	Participants in the study had difficulties with relationships in time (e.g., considering past, present, and future), with knowing when (i.e., reading time and knowing when appointments were), and knowing how long activities would last (judging time or knowing how long a spouse had been gone from the home). Spontaneous strategies to deal with temporal difficulties were used by some participants with varying degrees of success. Time aid interventions were initiated with all 5 participants; only 2 found them useful for assisting with knowing when and planning appointments. Difficulties related to "knowing how long" were not successfully addressed by the aids that were used by any of the participants.	Selecting people motivated for the intervention and able to participate in the interviews may have resulted in a "select" group of participants who are not similar to other people with dementia. The findings were clear and linked to the aims of the study; readers would benefit from more information about the analytic process. The conclusions were appropriately tenuous in terms of transferring the findings to others, and study limitations are identified.	People with dementia (especially with mild cognitive impairment) experiencing temporal difficulties with time orientation (i.e., knowing what time it is) and organizing time to make appointments may benefit from time aid interventions. Aids must be considered carefully so they are easy to understand and manipulate and difficult to alter by accident.

Nygård, L., & Johansson, M. (2001). The experience and management of temporality in five cases of dementia. *Scandinavian Journal of Occupational Therapy, 8*, 85–95.

(continued)

Qualitative Evidence: Routines

EVIDENCE TABLE: What is the evidence for the effectiveness of interventions designed to establish, modify, or maintain routines on the occupational performance, quality of life, health and wellness, and client and caregiver satisfaction of persons with Alzheimer's disease? (continued)

Author/Year	Study Objectives	Design and Participants	Findings	Trustworthiness/ Limitations	Implications for Occupational Therapy
Skovdahl, Kihlgren, A. L., & Kihlgren, 2003	The purposes of this study were to (a) better understand the types of interactions between caregivers and people with dementia that resulted in aggressive behavior and (b) identify the types of interactions with caregivers who reported problems with the behavior of aggressive residents and caregivers who did not report problems with the behavior of aggressive residents.	A phenomenological, hermeneutic approach was used. 2 participants considered the most difficult to work with were selected from different units for residents with dementia. The units were selected on the basis of previous reports of satisfaction with ability to cope with patient aggressiveness (1 unit satisfied and 1 not). Showering routine was videotaped 6×, 3× per patient. Each videotaped sequence was 20–35 min long with either 1 or 2 caregivers and 1 patient participating.	One finding related to the negative interactions that occurred when caregivers persisted in following a routine even when negative outcomes (resident agitation and aggression) were occurring. The authors described this as "being trapped in routines, where residents and caregivers remained in a negative interaction" (p. 895). It appeared that the focus was on completing the daily routine task of showering, rather than focusing on the residents' expressions and responses. The authors suggested that routines can become rituals that are followed without reflection or the possibility for adjustment.	The authors provided a clear presentation of the findings and their interpretations of them going from description to more interpretative analyses. The use of 2 authors in the analytic process further adds to the strength of the information. It is, however, difficult to draw solid conclusions because only 2 residents from 2 different units are included.	The focus on how tasks are completed implies that routines should not be adhered to without reflection on the responses of the care recipient. Occupational therapists with a focus on client-centered practice could facilitate consideration of staff versus patient routines, and whose needs are given highest priority. Caregivers might benefit from learning strategies to involve people with dementia in care routines in ways that share power. Occupational therapists could be involved in caregiver education related to client-centered practice and the completion of morning care routines that are responsive to needs of the clients.

Skovdahl, K., Kihlgren, A. L., & Kihlgren, M. (2003). Dementia and aggressiveness: Video recorded morning care from different care units. *Journal of Clinical Nursing, 12*, 888–898.

EVIDENCE TABLE: What is the effect of environmental-based interventions (e.g., Montessori and Snoezelen) on performance, affect, and behavior in both the home and institutions for people with Alzheimer's disease?

Author/Year	Study Objectives	Level/Design/ Participants	Intervention and Outcome Measures	Results	Study Limitations	Implications for Occupational Therapy
Chung & Lai, 2006	The objective was to examine the efficacy of Snoezelen (or multisensory stimulation) for older people with dementia and their caregivers.	Level I Systematic review	Articles chosen were RCTs or quasi-RCTs in which Snoezelen or multisensory program was used as an intervention for older persons with dementia.	The results of the 5 studies included in the review indicate that there is not evidence showing the efficacy of Snoezelen for dementia.	Meta-analyses could not be performed because of the limited number of trials and different study methods of the available trials.	This review found that there is no evidence showing the efficacy of Snoezelen for dementia. There is a need for more reliable and sound research-based evidences to inform and justify the use of Snoezelen in dementia care.
Chung, J. C. C., & Lai, C. K. Y. (2002). Snoezelen for dementia. *Cochrane Database of Systematic Reviews, 4*, CD003152 doi:10.1002/14651858.CD003152						
Dooley & Hinojosa, 2004	The objective was to examine the extent to which adherence to occupational therapy recommendations derived from individualized assessment would increase the quality of life of people with AD and to decrease the burden felt by persons caring for them in the community.	Level I Randomized, 2-group pretest–posttest Participants 40 people with possible or probable AD (16 men, 24 women, mean age 77) and their 40 caregivers (8 men, 32 women)	Intervention The intervention group received one 30-min session in their homes in which the occupational therapist explained recommendations for client and caregiver. Caregiver approach strategies based on the results of baseline measurements included structuring a daily routine, involving client in chores, cueing to break down tasks, giving directions 1 step at a time, suggesting activities to the client when unoccupied, and cueing to use visual cues and adaptive equipment. In the control group, caregivers were mailed a report of occupational therapy recommendations based on the results of baseline measures. Outcome Measures *At baseline and follow-up 1–6 mo later:* ▪ AIF ▪ Performance-based test of common IADLs	Caregivers in the treatment group followed 65.1% of the 5 most important recommended strategies. Comparison of baseline to follow-up measures indicated a significant difference in quality of life for clients, increased positive affect, and increased independence in self-care.	There was inconsistency of when caregivers were able to complete the follow-up assessments, and this inconsistency may have influenced the accuracy of the results, particularly for those in the treatment group.	Brief occupational therapy interventions can be effective when directed at improving the quality of life of persons with dementia. Interventions such as cueing to break down tasks, structuring daily routines, and suggesting activities to engage the client can assist in improving the client's affect, as well as improving independence in ADLs.

(continued)

Environmental Interventions

EVIDENCE TABLE: What is the effect of environmental-based interventions (e.g., Montessori and Snoezelen) on performance, affect, and behavior in both the home and institutions for people with Alzheimer's disease? *(continued)*

Author/Year	Study Objectives	Level/Design/ Participants	Intervention and Outcome Measures	Results	Study Limitations	Implications for Occupational Therapy
Dooley & Hinojosa, 2004 *(cont.)*			■ AAL–AD: Objective measure of quality of life rate by caregiver PSMS: self-care status measure done by caregiver			

Dooley, N. R., & Hinojosa, J. (2004). Improving quality of life for persons with Alzheimer's disease and their family caregivers: Brief occupational therapy intervention. *American Journal of Occupational Therapy, 58*, 561–569.

Author/Year	Study Objectives	Level/Design/ Participants	Intervention and Outcome Measures	Results	Study Limitations	Implications for Occupational Therapy
Kovach, Taneli, Dohearty, Schlidt, Cashin, & Silva-Smith, 2004	The objective was to test the effectiveness of the Balancing Arousal Controls Excesses (BACE) intervention in decreasing agitation in residents of long-term care with moderate or severe dementia.	Level I RCT double-blinded Participants *n* = 78 Moderate or severe dementia in 13 long-term-care facilities (intervention = 36 control = 42; men = 7, women = 71) Men = 7 of 78/9% Women = 71 of 78/91%	Intervention BACE, which controls the daily schedule to balance between the times a person is in high-arousal states and low-arousal states. ■ Phase 1 (assessment) every 15 min from 8:00 a.m.–8:00 p.m. on 1 day ■ Phase 2 (diagnose and plan a correction of the arousal imbalance) the day after Phase 1 to configure a new daily activity schedule ■ Phase 3 (nursing staff implemented new activity schedule and the research assistants assessed persons state of arousal and agitation every 15 min for 12 hr) within 7 days of Phase 1 The control group experienced usual care. For duration, see above (Range of stay was 1–97 mo—mean length of stay was 30.2 mo). Outcome Measures ■ Arousal States in Dementia scale ■ Wisconsin Agitation Intensity Parameters (visual analog scale)	The majority of participants' days were spent in a high level of arousal. There were no significant correlations between agitation and the amount of time spent in high arousal, minimal arousal, or disengaged. The mean agitation score for the control group stayed the same from pretest to posttest, the mean in the intervention group changed from 38.97 to 30.54 (*p* < .001). 30 of the 36 respondents in the treatment group had a decrease in agitation from pretest to posttest ranging from 1.91 points to 30.55 points. Agitation scores decreased significantly from pretesting to posttesting during the arousal imbalance time periods from the BACE intervention group (*p* = .04). There were no significant interaction effects in the 3 repeated measure ANCOVAs run using the 3 models, indicating that differences in agitation between the BACE intervention group and the control group were not dependent on whether the person was moderately or severely	A limited number of participants met eligibility requirements. Observation measures were subjective, and actions may have been misinterpreted by the researchers. The change in agitation behavior could have been a result of interaction or change in activity.	Occupational therapy could use the BACE intervention in settings such as long-term care or skilled nursing facilities to attempt to balance clients' states of arousal to decrease their agitation levels. The BACE intervention is low cost, simple, and nontechnological and could be implemented in community settings such as churches and adult day programs. The BACE intervention, based on the results of this study, seems to provide an effective treatment for and prevention of agitation.

cognitively impaired, whether the person slept a lot or a little during the day, or whether the person had retained or lost verbal skills.

Kovach, C. R., Taneli, Y., Dohearty, P., Schlidt, A. M., Cashin, S., & Silva-Smith, A. L. (2004). Effect of the BACE intervention on agitation of people with dementia. *Gerontologist, 44,* 797–806.

		Intervention		
Nolan, Mathews, & Harrison, 2001	The objective was to determine the effect of placing 2 external memory aids outside participants' bedrooms.	**Level IV** Single participant design multiple baseline **Participants** *N* = 3 women patients	A baseline of 17 to 21 observations was completed with each participant before the intervention of external memory aids were given. A laminated yellow card with a statement indicating who lived in the room was taped to the participant's door ("This is Mary's Room"). A portrait of the participant as a young adult was enlarged and attached to the back of the memory box outside the participant's room. A direct observation technique was used requiring 2 observers to affirm that the participant had successfully identified their room. Intervention was completed by daytime hospital staff, 5 days/wk for 2 mo in a SCU. **Outcome Measure** Successful location of room by participant	Baseline performance of room finding was low for all 3 participants. All 3 participants improved during the intervention phase. Mrs. A began at a baseline performance of room finding at 24% and increased to 80% during intervention. Mrs. B found her room 52% of the time at baseline and 100% of the time during intervention. Mrs. C went from 26% of room finding at baseline to 75% during intervention. Thus, there was > 50% mean increase in participants' ability to accurately locate their rooms after the intervention.	A larger sample should be used to ensure the accuracy of the results. The use of external memory aids in the form of signs with individual's name and portrait-like photographs can be used in either the clinical or community-based practice settings of occupational therapy. Displaying photographs and attaching a sign to a door is a low-cost and simple intervention that appears to increase the probability of older adults with severe AD successfully locating their nursing home bedroom. A patient's ability to navigate their environment is important in the completion of many activities of daily living and IADLs.

Nolan, B., Mathews, R., & Harrison, M. (2001). Using external memory aids to increase room finding by older adults with dementia. *American Journal of Alzheimer's Disease and Other Dementias, 16,* 251–254.

(continued)

Environmental Interventions

EVIDENCE TABLE: What is the effect of environmental-based interventions (e.g., Montessori and Snoezelen) on performance, affect, and behavior in both the home and institutions for people with Alzheimer's disease? *(continued)*

Author/Year	Study Objectives	Level/Design/ Participants	Intervention and Outcome Measures	Results	Study Limitations	Implications for Occupational Therapy
Opie, Rosewarne, & O'Connor, 1999	This paper provides a systematic review of research findings published between 1989 and 1998 concerning nonpharmacological strategies to alleviate behavioral disturbances in elderly people with dementia.	<u>Level I</u> Systematic review 43 articles included in the review.	<u>Intervention</u> Interventions studied were grouped into the following categories: ■ Changes to the physical environment ■ Activity programs ■ Exposure to music, voice, and language ■ Massage and aroma therapy ■ Light therapy, multidisciplinary teams, and carer education	43 studies met inclusion criteria and were conducted in a variety of settings. Validity ratings were as follows: 1 strong, 15 moderate, and 27 weak. The results of the review indicate that there is evidence to support the efficacy of activity programs, music, behavior therapy, light therapy, carer education, and changes to the physical environment. The evidence in favor of multidisciplinary teams, massage, and aromatherapy is inconclusive.	Most of the studies included in this research had limited rigor. Only 1 study reviewed had a high validity rating. Limitations of the studies included small numbers of participants, inadequate descriptions of study participants, imprecise data collection methods, high attrition rates, and insufficient statistical analysis	There is a need for more rigorous research in the area of nonpharmacological interventions with persons with AD. The authors found that research supports the use of activity programs, music, behavior therapy, light therapy, carer education, and changes to the environment.

Opie, J., Rosewarne, R., & O'Connor, D. (1999). The efficacy of psychosocial approaches to behaviour disorders in dementia: A systematic literature review. *Australian and New Zealand Journal of Psychiatry, 33*, 789–799.

| Orsulic-Jeras, Judge, & Camp 2000 | The objective was to examine the effects of Montessori-based activities programming on various forms of engagement exhibited by residents with advanced dementia in a long-term-care facility. | <u>Level II</u>
Within-participant, nonrandomized control with regular unit programming and Montessori-based programming

<u>Participants</u>
n = 16 with advanced dementia (men = 2, women = 14) | <u>Intervention</u>
The intervention was Montessori-based programming that included individual activities and 2 small group activities (Memory Bingo and Group Sorting). Individual activities consisted of aesthetically pleasing materials taken from the everyday environment of the resident. The control group had regular unit programming that included large group (storytelling, trivia, exercise and current events), small group (hand massage, aromatherapy, | Substantially more constructive engagement was observed during Montessori-based programming than during regular programming (*p* < .001). Residents showed less passive engagement in Montessori-based programming than in regular programming (*p* < .03). Although instances of nonengagement and self-engagement were not often observed during the activity periods, when nonengagement and self-engagement were observed they were almost exclusively during regular | The study was conducted in only 1 facility that promoted small group activities, limiting the generalization to facilities solely performing large group practices. Small sample size and lack of randomization are further limitations. | Montessori-based activities can be used in both the institutional and community-based settings. Occupational therapists should continue to research the efficacy of Montessori-based programming in order to potentially provide this type of programming to the ever-increasing geriatric population. Because of the low cost associated with implementing Montessori-based programs, this can be another tool used by occupational therapists, with minimal costs to the |

Author/Year	Objective	Level/Design/Participants	Intervention/Outcome Measures	Results	Comments/Limitations
			and tai chi), and individual activities (puzzles and individual time with staff). Both groups took place twice per week for 15–20 min per session over a period of 9 mo. **Outcome Measures** ■ Constructive Engagement, Passive Engagement, Nonengagement, and Self-Engagement Measure— ■ Affect Rating Scale—Assess instances of pleasure, anger, anxiety/fear, and sadness	programming, not during Montessori programming. Pleasure scores were significantly higher during Montessori programming than during regular unit activities ($p < .001$). Anxiety was higher during regular programming ($p < .003$). Neither anger nor sadness were observed in many of the participants, but when they did occur, they were almost exclusively seen during regular programming, not during Montessori-based programming.	facility. A training manual is available to help practitioners, students, and family members create and implement Montessori-based activities. However, minimal research has been conducted on the effects of Montessori-based programming on people with advanced dementia. Therefore, consideration should be taken when deciding whether or not to implement the program.

Orsulic-Jeras, S., Judge, K., & Camp, C. (2000). Montessori-based activities for long-term care residents with advanced dementia: Effects on engagement and affect. *Gerontologist, 40,* 107–111.

Author/Year	Objective	Level/Design/Participants	Intervention	Results	Comments/Limitations
Swanson, Maas, & Buckwalter, 1994	The objective was to compare the effects of an SCU with that of a traditional (integrated) unit for persons with AD.	**Level II** Nonrandomized control trial **Participants** $N = 22$ with middle stage AD (13 in SCU and 9 in control conditions; men = 20, women = 2)	**Intervention** Intervention entailed use of a self-contained unit for ambulatory AD residents, designed to segregate AD residents from nondemented residents and to allow unrestricted safe wandering on the unit. Sensory stimuli were controlled by keeping traffic and noise at a minimum, by playing soothing music, and quiet, yet pleasant décor of designs, textures, and colors. Each staff member received 40 classroom hours and 40 supervised clinical practicum hours and was assigned to the SCU unit and did not rotate on to other units. Control AD residents were integrated into the non-SCU traditional units.	There was no difference on performance on cognitive/noncognitive measures and functional abilities as measured by ADAS and FAC respectively. Both the SCU and control participants demonstrated a decline in cognitive ability following the opening of the SCU. Catastrophic reactions decreased significantly for the SCU group compared with the non-SCU group as measured by individual incident.	The extended time frame may result in maturation of the disease process. Reliability and validity were not established for the individual incident and FAC, which were developed by the authors. The sample size was small, and the interventions were performed in 1 facility. While the study began as a RCT, attrition due to death made this difficult. The study above indicated that while participants on the SCU demonstrated better behavior than their counterparts on traditional units, there were no statistical differences between the 2 groups. Occupational therapists and students can contribute to the body of knowledge on this subject area by performing evidence-based research. Additional studies are needed in order to increase the efficacy of SCUs for individuals with AD.

(continued)

EVIDENCE TABLE: What is the effect of environmental-based interventions (e.g., Montessori and Snoezelen) on performance, affect, and behavior in both the home and institutions for people with Alzheimer's disease? *(continued)*

Author/Year	Study Objectives	Level/Design/ Participants	Intervention and Outcome Measures	Results	Study Limitations	Implications for Occupational Therapy
Swanson, Maas, & Buckwalter, 1994 *(cont.)*			Both groups participated 24-hr/day, 4 mo before and 4 mo after the opening of the SCU. Outcome Measures ■ ADAS: Cognitive and non-cognitive functioning and behavioral dysfunctions ■ GDS: Cognitive status of individuals with AD ■ FAC: Self-care, cognitive status ■ Individual incident: Catastrophic and other disruptive behaviors			

Swanson, E., Maas, M., & Buckwalter, K. (1994). Alzheimer's residents cognitive and functional measures. *Clinical Nursing, 3,* 27–41.

| Whall, Black, Groh, Yankou, Kupferschmid, & Foster, 1997 | The objective was to examine the effect of natural environments on agitated and aggressive behavior during nursing care procedures (showering) in late-stage dementia patients. | Level II Nonrandomized control trial 2-group Participants $N = 31$ with late-stage AD dementia or a mixture of AD with multi-infarct dementia in 2 nursing homes (intervention = 15; control = 16; men = 4, women = 27) | Intervention Natural experience: After baseline, the treatment group was bathed in a shower room that featured recorded songs of birds, sounds of babbling brooks, and the sounds of other small animals. Also, large bright pictures were coordinated with the tapes. A third natural element was to provide food each patient preferred and that was compatible with their individual dietary restrictions. The control group received usual care at baseline and 2 subsequent baths 1 wk apart. Outcome Measure Agitation and aggression (modified CMAI) | The mean length of the shower bath in both groups was 7–10 min. Agitation decreased significantly in the treatment group compared with the control group. There was a significant decline in agitated behavior from baseline to Treatment 1 ($p < .02$) and baseline to Treatment 2 ($p < .004$). However, between Treatment 1 and Treatment 2 there was no significant difference. Physical aggression decreased over time in the treatment group, but was not significantly decreased. | Lack of randomization of the trial and small sample size limit generalizability. | This intervention is beneficial for occupational therapists because it is a low-cost way to decrease agitated and aggressive behavior without the use of medications or restraints. This study indicates that using a natural environment simulation in various settings would improve the relationship between the caregiver and the individual. Because of the low cost, this type of intervention could be implemented in institutional facilities, community-based settings, or in a home setting. |

Whall, A. L., Black, M. E., Groh, C. J., Yankou, D. J., Kupferschmid, B. J., & Foster, M. L. (1997). The effect of natural environments upon agitation and aggression in late stage dementia patients. *American Journal of Alzheimer's Diseases, 12*, 216–220.

EVIDENCE TABLE: What is the effectiveness of intervention designed to modify the activity demands of the occupations of self-care, leisure, and social participation for persons with dementia? (Activity Demands)

Author/Year	Study Objectives	Level/Design/ Participants	Intervention and Outcome Measures	Results	Study Limitations	Implications for Occupational Therapy
Coyne & Hoskins, 1997	The objective was to determine the short- and long-term efficacy of directed verbal prompts and positive reinforcement on the level of eating independence of elderly nursing home residents with dementia.	Level I Randomized 2-group Pretest–posttest design with repeated measures and random selection Participants 24 women (age range 68–96) diagnosed with dementia living in a dementia-unit of a skilled nursing facility	Intervention The intervention group was provided with directed verbal prompts at 1-min intervals and positive reinforcement on completing each step of the eating cycle to promote independence in eating during meals in the dining room setting. The prompts were standardized and were given by the researcher or research assistant. The treatment took place during 3 daily meals for 3 consecutive days. Outcome Measures Level of eating independence scale on the basis of the Klein-Bell ADL scale administered as pretest and 2 posttests.	A significant difference was noted between the control and intervention groups on task performance with solid and liquid foods indicating greater independence for those receiving the intervention. No significant difference was noted between groups for frequency of completed task cycles of eating.	All of the participants in the study were women, which limits generalizability. Sample size was small. The study was limited to 1 dementia unit.	The results indicated that verbal prompts and positive reinforcement increase the eating independence of persons with dementia and therefore the diagnosis should not preclude the possibility that these individuals may regain some lost skills used in eating. However, these strategies do not necessarily increase the frequency of completed task cycles of eating. Results of this study indicate that future research could be done by occupational therapy professionals to determine the effectiveness of these strategies with a larger and more representative sample as well as with other ADLs.

Coyne, M. L., & Hoskins, L. (1997). Improving eating behaviors in dementia using behavioral strategies. *Clinical Nursing Research, 6*, 275–290.

| Dooley & Hinojosa, 2004 | The objective was to examine the extent to which adherence to occupational therapy recommendations derived from individualized assessment would increase the quality of life of people with AD and decrease the burden felt by people caring for them in the community. | Level I

Randomized
2-group
pretest–posttest

Participants

40 people with possible or probable AD (16 men, 24 women, mean age = 77) and their 40 caregivers (8 men, 32 women) | Intervention

The intervention group received one 30-min session in their homes in which the occupational therapist explained recommendations for client and caregiver. Caregiver approach strategies on the basis of the results of baseline measurements included: structuring a | Caregivers in the treatment group followed 65.1% of the 5 most important recommended strategies. Comparison of baseline to follow-up measures indicated a significant difference in quality of life for clients, increased positive affect, and increased independence in self-care. | There was inconsistency of when caregivers were able to complete the follow-up assessments, and this inconsistency may have influenced the accuracy of the results, particularly for those in the treatment group. | Brief occupational therapy interventions can be effective when directed at improving the quality of life of persons with dementia. Interventions such as cueing to break down tasks, structuring daily routines, and suggesting activities to engage the client can assist in improving the client's affect, as well as |

improving independence in activities of daily living.

daily routine, involving client in chores, cueing to break down tasks, giving directions 1 step at a time, suggesting activities to the client when unoccupied, and cueing to use visual cues and adaptive equipment.

In the control group, caregivers were mailed a report of occupational therapy recommendations based on the results of baseline measures

Outcome Measures
(at baseline and follow-up 1–6 mo later):
- AIF: Performance-based test of common IADLs
- AAL-AD: Objective measure of quality of life rate by caregiver
- PSMS: Self-care status measure reported by caregiver

Dooley, N. R., & Hinojosa, J. (2004). Improving quality of life for persons with Alzheimer's disease and their family caregivers: Brief occupational therapy intervention. *American Journal of Occupational Therapy, 58,* 561–569.

| Graff, Vernooij-Dassen, Thijssen, Dekker, Hoefnagels, & Rikkert, 2006 | The objective was to determine the effectiveness of community-based occupational therapy on daily functioning of patients with dementia and the sense of competence of their caregivers. | Level I
Single blind RCT

Participants
135 people age ≥ 65 with mild to moderate dementia who were living in the community and attended a memory clinic and day clinic, as well as their caregivers | Intervention
The intervention group received 10 1-hr sessions of occupational therapy in their homes over 5 wk. 4 sessions consisted of identifying activities to focus improvement on and the next 6 involved educating clients on compensatory and environmental strategies to improve ADLs performance. | At 6-wk, the intervention group showed a significant difference in improvement in functioning in daily activities compared to the control group. 84% of the intervention group had a clinically relevant improvement on the process outcome of the AMPS. At 12 wk, the intervention group still demonstrated better daily functioning. | The researchers were only able to do a single blind study because the clients/caregivers were aware of which therapy they received and therapists were not able to be blinded either. Another limitation is that the researchers selected their participants from outpatient clinics instead of a variety of | The results of this study indicate the value of community-based occupational therapy interventions for persons with mild to moderate dementia. Effects in improved daily functioning through community-based cognitive and behavioral interventions twice weekly over a period of 10 wk were still present at 12 wk after treatment, which justifies implementation of |

(continued)

EVIDENCE TABLE: What is the effectiveness of intervention designed to modify the activity demands of the occupations of self-care, leisure, and social participation for persons with dementia? (Activity Demands) (continued)

Author/Year	Study Objectives	Level/Design/ Participants	Intervention and Outcome Measures	Results	Study Limitations	Implications for Occupational Therapy
Graff, Vernooij-Dassen, Thijssen, Dekker, Hoefnagels, & Rikkert, 2006 (cont.)			<u>Outcome Measures</u> ▪ Process scale of the AMPS ▪ Performance scale of the IDDD		settings such as general practices, which would have given a more representative sample of this population.	this intervention. Because dementia is a progressive condition, compensatory strategies are one of the main ways to keep these clients functioning independently for as long as possible.

Graff, M. J. L., Vernooij-Dassen, M. J. M., Thijssen, M., Dekker, J., Hoefnagels, W. H. L., & Rikkert, M. G. M. (2006). Community-based occupational therapy for patients with dementia and their caregivers: Randomised controlled trial. *British Medical Journal, 333,* 1196–1201.

Author/Year	Study Objectives	Level/Design/ Participants	Intervention and Outcome Measures	Results	Study Limitations	Implications for Occupational Therapy
Kolanowski, 2001	The objective was to test the utility of theory-based activity selection for treating behaviors commonly exhibited by people with dementia.	<u>Level I</u> Randomized Crossover experimental design <u>Participants</u> 10 residents with a diagnosis of dementia from 2 nursing homes	<u>Intervention</u> The 10 nursing home residents served as their own control in this cross-over experimental pilot study. Using the NEO Five Factor Inventory to assess premorbid personality and interest style, participants were engaged in activities suited to their style of interest and skill level. Control activities were selected from those opposite to participants' style of interest. <u>Outcomes Measures</u> ▪ Positive and negative moods were measured using the Philadelphia Geriatric Center Affect Rating Scale and the Dementia Mood Picture Test ▪ Dementia behaviors were measured using the CMAI ▪ Cognitive ability was measured using the Folstein MMSE ▪ Physical ability was measured using the physical capacity subscale of the Psychogeriatric Dependency Rating Scale	Displays of positive affect were significantly higher during treatment than control, but there was no statistical difference in displays of negative affect between conditions. No significant difference in mood following conditions or difference in dementia behaviors between conditions were reported.	Sample size was too small.	This study emphasizes the value of client-centered and occupation-based interventions for individuals with dementia.

Kolanowski, A. (2001). Capturing interests: Therapeutic recreation activities for persons with dementia. *Therapeutic Recreation Journal, 35,* 220–235.

Study	Objective	Design/Participants	Intervention	Results	Comments
Rogers, Holm, Burgio, Granieri, Hsu, & Hardin, 1999	This study examined the effectiveness of a behavioral rehabilitation intervention for improving the performance of morning care ADLs of nursing home residents with dementia.	**Level III** 3 × 3 design (condition × ADL category) **Participants** 84 participants (58 women and 26 men; mean age = 82) with a dementia diagnosis and dressing disability must remain in the facility for > 3 mo	**Intervention** Usual care and a period of naturalistic observation was followed by the intervention of skill elicitation, which in turn was followed by individualized behavioral interventions for habit training to reinforce skills and improve functional gains. **Outcome Measure** Observational information of ADLs was recorded using the Portable Computer Systems for Observational Research (Observe) software.	The results demonstrated behavioral rehabilitative care significantly improved ADL participation among the residents with dementia and their caregivers. Compared with usual care, skill elicitation participants exhibited increased independence in performing dressing tasks, increased participation in assisted dressing, decreased disruptive behaviors, and increased appropriate requests for help. Although the assistance provided by caregivers decreased, caregiver time to participate in the program increased.	Outcome measures were based only on observations rather than standardized measures. A control group was lacking.	It can be extrapolated that behavioral rehabilitative intervention in occupational therapy can significantly improve patient outcomes in the areas of independence in performing dressing subtasks, increased participation in assisted dressing, a decreased incidence of disruptive behaviors, and increased incidence in appropriate requests for help with ADLs for nursing home residents.

Rogers, J. C., Holm, M. B., Burgio, L. D., Granieri, E., Hsu, C., & Hardin, J. M. (1999). Improving morning care routines of nursing home residents with dementia. *Journal of the American Geriatrics Society, 47,* 1049–1057.

Study	Objective	Design/Participants	Intervention	Results	Comments
Spector, Thorgrtimsen, Woods, Royan, Davies, Butterworth, et al., 2003	The objective was to determine whether cognitive stimulation improves cognition and quality of life.	**Level I** RCT Single blinded Multicenter **Participants** 201 participants diagnosed with dementia (115 receiving CST and 86 controls)	**Intervention** CST was the intervention provided to participants at residential homes or day centers. Intervention was provided in groups 45 min 2×/wk for 7 wk. Control participants underwent their usual activities while group therapy was in progress **Outcomes Measures** ■ MMSE ■ ADAS-Cog ■ QoL-AD	CST significantly improved cognitive function compared with usual activities as measured by MMSE and ADAS-Cog. There were also significantly higher scores on the QoL-AD for the intervention group. There were no differences, however, on communication, functional ability, anxiety, or depression.	There was significant variation between centers and the improvement of cognitive function scores.	This study demonstrated the potential for using CST, including adapting the level of activity based on the individual's ability. Cognitive therapy can be used as means to improve cognitive function and improve quality of life; however, it is important to consider the variability among patients with the diagnosis of dementia of the AD type.

Spector, A., Thorgrtimsen, L., Woods, B., Royan, L., Davies, S., Butterworth, M., et al. (2003). Efficacy of an evidence-based cognitive stimulation therapy program for people with dementia. *British Journal of Psychiatry, 183,* 248–254.

(continued)

Activity Demands

EVIDENCE TABLE: What is the effectiveness of intervention designed to modify the activity demands of the occupations of self-care, leisure, and social participation for persons with dementia? *(Activity Demands) (continued)*

Author/Year	Study Objectives	Level/Design/ Participants	Intervention and Outcome Measures	Results	Study Limitations	Implications for Occupational Therapy
Watson & Green, 2006	The objective was to systematically review nursing literature on interventions used to decrease feeding difficulty in individuals with AD.	<u>Level I</u> Systematic review 13 studies were included in the review	<u>Intervention</u> This systematic review included quasi-experimental, retrospective, case comparison, and RCTs that used changes in meal preparation and delivery, addition of music to meal time, incorporation of verbal prompts, and environmental modification.	All 13 studies reported positive outcomes and included changes in activity demands (meal presentation and verbal prompts by different carers) as well as environmental changes (use of music and change of dining setting).	There were no standardized interventions across the studies. No study reported the use of power analysis. Suspected reporting bias limited this review. Only 1 RCT was included in the review. Many studies did not account for confounding factors. Sample sizes were small.	Although high-quality evidence is limited, it appears that changes in meal presentation and consistent verbal prompts across carers, as well as changing the environment to improve eating behaviors (including the use of music), may be effective for older adults with dementia.

Watson, R., & Green, S. (2006). Feeding and dementia: A systematic literature review. *Journal of Advanced Nursing, 54,* 86–93.

EVIDENCE TABLE: What is the evidence for the effect of interventions to prevent falls in persons with dementia? Intervention approaches to consider include adaptation, remediation, prevention, and maintenance. Performance areas to examine include self-care, leisure, and social participation. (Client Factors)

Author/Year	Study Objectives	Level/Design/ Participants	Intervention and Outcome Measures	Results	Study Limitations	Implications for Occupational Therapy
Detweiler, Kim, & Taylor, 2005	The objective was to determine the effectiveness of having a intense fall-focused program provided by regular care providers.	Level III Nonrandomized control trial 1 group Pretest and posttest Participants 8 dementia patients with the highest fall incidence were chosen for the study.	Intervention 2 CNAs provided care on the day and evening shift to the residents on a consistent basis every day for intense fall-focused supervision. Included were in-services related to fall prevention and keeping participants occupied during the shift. Outcome Measures Number of falls	There was a statistically significant decrease in the number of falls during the intervention period. The total number of falls during baseline period was 112; during intervention period it was 62, and the mean reduction in fall number was 6.26. There was not difference in fall severity between baseline and intervention.	The total baseline and intervention period was limited. 1 of the CNAs left after the end of the study period. The 8 study participants lived scattered among other residents. The sample size was small.	Supervision and involvement in activity-based intervention may be effective in reducing the number of falls by high-risk dementia patients.

Detweiler, M. B., Kim, K. Y., & Taylor, B. Y. (2005). Focused supervision of high-risk fall dementia patients: A simple method to reduce fall incidence and severity. *American Journal of Alzheimer's Disease and Other Dementias, 20*, 97–104.

| Hauer, Becker, Lindemann, & Beyer, 2006 | The objective was to determine whether older cognitively impaired people benefit from physical training with regard to motor performance or fall risk reduction and to critically evaluate the methodological approach in RCTs. | Level I Systematic review Published RCTs from 1966 through 2004 that focused on people with cognitive impairment Literature search using Cochrane Central Register of controlled trials, MEDLINE, CINAHL, and GEROLIT published between 1993 and 2004 | Intervention Physical training for fall prevention for older adults with cognitive impairments living in a variety of settings was implemented. Outcome Measures Outcome measures included measurements of muscle strength, flexibility, and specific functional performances such as walking, postural control, global motor or functional performance scores (e.g., activities of daily living), physical activity, or falls/ fall-related outcomes. | The results of 11 RCTs indicate that the evidence for the effectiveness of physical training in patients with cognitive impairment is unclear. Training effects on motor performance and consequently on reduction of falls, when reported, were most often related to improvements in gait variables. | Dementia diagnosis was not performed. Screening tests did not give specific diagnoses. The review addressed cognitive impairment, not AD dementia specifically. Study samples were homogenous. Some articles had small sample sizes. Meta-analysis could not be performed because of the heterogeneity of studies. | This area is understudied, and further research is needed. Although conclusions are tentative, physical interventions such as gait, strengthening, balance, and flexibility training had a positive effect on gait variables and, therefore, indirectly may result in reduction of number of falls. Occupational therapists should embed features of these interventions in occupation-based programs. |

Hauer, K., Becker, C., Lindemann, U., & Beyer, N. (2006). Effectiveness of physical training on motor performance and fall prevention in cognitively impaired older persons: A systematic review. *American Journal of Physical Medicine and Rehabilitation, 85*, 847–857.

(continued)

Falls Prevention

EVIDENCE TABLE: What is the evidence for the effect of interventions to prevent falls in persons with dementia? Intervention approaches to consider include adaptation, remediation, prevention, and maintenance. Performance areas to examine include self-care, leisure, and social participation. (Client Factors) (continued)

Author/Year	Study Objectives	Level/Design/ Participants	Intervention and Outcome Measures	Results	Study Limitations	Implications for Occupational Therapy
Mackintosh & Sheppard, 2005	The objective was to assess the value and feasibility of a falls-prevention program for community-dwelling older people with moderate to severe levels of dementia and prevalent Italian background.	<u>Level III</u> Pretest–posttest single-group design <u>Participants</u> 64 community-dwelling participants who were ≥ 50, had a history of dementia, and were medically stable (21 women; 43 men)	Baseline assessments included medical history, medications, number of falls in the last 12 mo, and a falls-risk assessment. <u>Intervention</u> 15-mo falls-prevention program was embedded within a healthy lifestyle dementia respite program. Participants generally attended once per week, although occasionally they did so with greater frequency. <u>Outcome Measures</u> ■ Fall status (based on number of falls within past 12 mo at baseline and past 6 mo at follow-up) ■ MMSE ■ Berg Balance Scale ■ Aerobic capacity (6-min walk)	No significant differences in outcomes measured between baseline and 6-mo follow-up.	There was a high dropout rate because of a variety of reasons, including transfer to residential care and death, resulting in a small sample size. Feasibility of intervention indicated by authors, but *how* authors came to their conclusions was unclear. People who examined assessments also performed intervention.	More research needs to be conducted on this type of program, but limited evidence suggests a falls-prevention program embedded in respite day programs may be a useful model to prevent falls and decrease caregiver burden if transportation, language assistance, small group size, and individual supervision are available.

Mackintosh, S. F., & Sheppard, L. A. (2005). A pilot falls-prevention programme for older people with dementia from a predominantly Italian background. *Hong Kong Physiotherapy Journal, 23,* 20–26.

			Interventions		Comments	
Oliver, Connelly, Victor, Shaw, Whitehead, Genc, et al., 2007	The objective was to evaluate the evidence for strategies to prevent falls or fractures in residents in care homes and hospital inpatients and to investigate the effect of dementia and cognitive impairment.	Level I Systematic review Meta-analysis 43 RCTs Case-control studies focused on people with dementia/cognitive impairments published between 1982 and 2005	Studies were single- or multifaceted and included hip protector, removal of physical restraint, fall alarm, exercise, change in environment, calcium/vitamin D, medication review; in care home or hospital.	Multifaceted interventions moderately reduced rate of falls in hospital settings. Evidence was inconclusive for multifaceted intervention in care home setting and for single faceted interventions in hospital and care home settings. Results of meta-regressions to assess effect of dementia were insignificant.	There is likely recorder bias for outcomes measures in some studies included in the review. Multifaceted interventions were undefined. Authors believe RCT design is insufficient within same setting, leading to corruption of control group. Only 1 study focused on persons with dementia, and the authors made the assumption that if prevalence was not mentioned in article, the prevalence was ≥ 70%. Dementia and cognitive impairment were undefined.	Results of this meta-analysis suggest that evidence is inconclusive that multifaceted interventions are effective overall in reducing the rate of falls, with exception of hospital settings. Although the evidence is limited for people with dementia, occupational therapy professionals should participate in inclusion of such strategies in hospital settings where they are more likely to be effective.

Oliver, D., Connelly J. B., Victor, C. R., Shaw, F. E., Whitehead, A., Genc, Y., et al. (2007). Strategies to prevent falls and fractures in hospitals and effect of cognitive impairment: Systematic review and meta-analyses. *British Medical Journal, 334*(7584), 82

(continued)

Falls Prevention

EVIDENCE TABLE: What is the evidence for the effect of interventions to prevent falls in persons with dementia? Intervention approaches to consider include adaptation, remediation, prevention, and maintenance. Performance areas to examine include self-care, leisure, and social participation. (Client Factors) (continued)

Author/Year	Study Objectives	Level/Design/ Participants	Intervention and Outcome Measures	Results	Study Limitations	Implications for Occupational Therapy
Stenvall, Olofsson, Lundstroom, Englund, Borssén, Svensson, et al., 2007	This study evaluated whether a postoperative, multidisciplinary, intervention program—including systematic assessment and treatment of fall risk factors, active prevention, detection, and treatment of postoperative complications—could reduce inpatient falls and fall-related injuries after a femoral neck fracture.	_Level I_ RCT _Participants_ 199 participants age ≥ 70; 74 women, 125 men _Inclusion criteria:_ Patients with undisplaced femoral neck fracture, operated on with internal fixation. Patients with displaced fracture operated on with hemiarthroplasty. 36/199 patients with dementia. _Exclusion criteria:_ Patients with— ■ Rheumatoid arthritis ■ Severe hip osteoarthritis ■ Pathological fracture ■ Severe renal failure ■ Bedridden before fracture occurred	_Intervention_ Intervention group was in a hospital unit specializing in geriatric orthopedic patients. A multidisciplinary team (registered nurses, licensed practical nurses, physiotherapists, occupational therapists, dietitian, and geriatricians) received a 4-day course in caring, rehabilitation, teamwork, and medical knowledge, including sessions about how to prevent, detect, and treat various postoperative complications such as postoperative delirium and falls. All team members assessed patients within 24 hr of arrival. The team met for goal setting twice per week and provided active prevention, detection, treatment of postoperative rehabilitation with a focus on prevention, daily routine, and nutrition. Home visits were made by occupational therapists or physical therapists.	Intervention group had overall fewer number of falls distributed over fewer fallers, fewer number of serious injuries, and shorter overall hospital stay (28.0±17.9 days intervention compared with 38.0±40.6 days control). Fewer number of falls and fallers among people with dementia.	Fall registration was not blinded, according to group allocation. The study sample was small, particularly of people with dementia.	Although the sample of participants with dementia was small, results suggest that occupational therapy professionals should advocate for and be part of multidisciplinary, postoperative intervention programs during inpatient stays to reduce the number of falls and fall-related injuries following a femoral neck fracture. Occupational therapy professionals can particularly provide basic ADLs routine training with particular attention to fall risk factors. There appears to be very little increased costs associated with this intervention program, with exception of education hours.

The control group also was on a specialist orthopedic geriatric unit, received usual care, team goals, and assessment once per week.

Outcome Measures
- AIS
- Maximum injury connected with each incident recorded
- MMSE
- OBS Scale
- GDS-15

Stenvall, M., Olofsson, B., Lundstroom, M., Englund, U., Borssén, B., Svensson, O., et al. (2007). A multidisciplinary, multifactorial intervention program reduces postoperative falls and injuries after femoral neck fracture. *Osteoporos International, 18,* 167–175.

EVIDENCE TABLE: What is the effectiveness of educational and supportive strategies for caregivers of persons with dementia on the ability to maintain participation in that role? *(Contexts)*

Author/Year	Study Objectives	Level/Design/ Participants	Intervention and Outcome Measures	Results	Study Limitations	Implications for Occupational Therapy
Acton & Kang, 2001	The objective was to evaluate, using meta-analytic techniques, those intervention strategies (support group, education, psychoeducation, counseling, respite care, and multicomponent) designed to help caregivers cope with the burden of caregiving.	<u>Level I</u> Meta-analysis 24 studies were included in the analysis.	<u>Intervention</u> This meta-analysis included studies that tested an intervention to reduce the burden of caregiving (support group, education, psychoeducation, counseling, and respite care). 17 of the studies reported using both a treatment and a control group, and 7 reported a 1-group pretest–posttest design. <u>Outcome Measures</u> ▪ Burden Interview ▪ Burden Scale ▪ Other burden scales designed for each study	Only 2 of the 27 treatments had a statistically significant positive effect on burden (respite intervention and multicomponent intervention), but pooled analyses showed no significant effect. The multicomponent intervention category appeared to reduce subjective burden, although only 1 study showed significant reduction. Respite care did not significantly reduce burden in situations where caregivers did not understand how to use the services or waited until crisis situations before seeking services.	Burden as a measure of caregiver outcomes was not well defined, with some studies measuring objective and others subjective indicators. The effect of interventions that were evaluated by 2 different measures (Burden Interview and Burden Scale) were pooled, which may have provided ambiguous results. Studies varied in participant size from 11 to 180. No other descriptions of study participants were included in the meta-analysis.	An intervention for caregivers may affect some of the tasks or time spent, but the caregiver remains responsible for the care, and thus, the intervention is unlikely to change the perception of responsibility, one of the indicators most often analyzed in burden measures. Although the quality of evidence is limited, it appears that a combination of supportive and educational strategies is of most use to caregivers. Rather than blanketing caregivers with a variety of interventions, these interventions should be implemented at the times they are needed, thus increasing the likelihood of better outcomes. Burden may not be the best outcome to demonstrate the effectiveness of caregiver interventions.

Acton, G. J., & Kang, J. (2001). Interventions to reduce the burden of caregiving for an adult with dementia: A meta-analysis. *Research in Nursing and Health, 24,* 349–360.

| Bank, Argüelles, Rubert, Eisdorfer, & Czaja, 2006 | The objective was to demonstrate the use of technology for conducting telephone-based support groups in ethnically diverse dementia caregivers. | Level III 1 group, nonrandomized, survey after intervention Participants 41 White American and Cuban American dementia caregivers participation at the Miami site of the REACH program Participants were predominantly women (76%) and Cuban-American (54%). 18 were wives and 10 were husbands of the care recipients. 11 were either daughters or daughters-in-law, and 2 were sisters of care recipients. The mean age of care recipients was 80 yr. | Intervention The computer-telephone integrated system (CTIS) system, an information network that relies on computer-telephone technology (screen phones allow both voice and text data to be sent and received during interactive session). All participants received in-home, family therapy sessions during the first 12 mo of the study. In addition, CTIS phones were placed in each participant's home. Telephone support group sessions with a maximum of 6 caregivers, facilitated by a study-certified therapist, and approx 1 hr. in length were held bimonthly at the beginning of the intervention period and then monthly thereafter for 18 mo. Non-Hispanic White caregivers participated in English-language groups, and Hispanic caregivers participated in Spanish-language groups. Outcome Measures A Support Group Questionnaire was developed for this study. | The mean number of sessions attended was 7.1. 81% of participants found the group "valuable." There was no statistically significant difference between White and Cuban-American caregivers. 73% of individuals reported their participation had increased their knowledge and skills as caregivers; 70% reported participation had increased their knowledge about memory disorders like AD; 68% reported their participation had increased their knowledge of community resources for caregivers; 62% reported participation had improved their relationships with members of their family; and 51% reported participation in the telephone support group had made them more willing to attend a support group in the community. | Sample size was small. The effect of the telephone support intervention by itself on psychosocial outcomes could not be examined because all components of the CTIS system were delivered to all participants. Only self-reported data were obtained, and they were not verified. | Occupational therapy professionals should consider enhancing their service with telephone-based support for caregivers, particularly in rural areas or where caregivers do not have easy access to care centers. Such a system could serve to follow-up on in-home therapy. Occupational therapy professionals' psychosocial education prepares them well to serve as co-facilitators for such support groups as part of an interdisciplinary team. Occupational therapy professionals can particularly focus on the ADL challenges faced by caregivers and assist them in identifying strategies with which they may feel and be successful. |

Bank, A. L., Argüelles, S., Rubert, M., Eisdorfer, C., & Czaja, S. J. (2006). The value of telephone support groups among ethnically diverse caregivers of persons with dementia. *Gerontologist, 46*, 134–138

(continued)

EVIDENCE TABLE: What is the effectiveness of educational and supportive strategies for caregivers of persons with dementia on the ability to maintain participation in that role? (Contexts) (continued)

Author/Year	Study Objectives	Level/Design/ Participants	Intervention and Outcome Measures	Results	Study Limitations	Implications for Occupational Therapy
Brodaty, Green, & Koschera, 2003	The objective was to review published reports on interventions for caregivers of persons with dementia, excluding respite care, and provide recommendation for clinicians.	Level I Meta-analysis 30 studies (involving 2,040 caregivers) reporting on 34 interventions were included in the review.	Intervention Interventions included counseling of carers, education, family counseling, patient involvement, support groups/programs, stress management, and training. Outcome Measures Primary outcome measures were psychological morbidity (GHQ, Hamilton Depressions Scale, Brief Symptom Inventory, Self Rating Depression Scale, Hopkins Symptom Checklist, CES-D, and Positive and Negative Affect Scale) and burden (Burden Interview, Rankin Scale, Caregivers Hassles Scale, Screen for Caregiver Burden).	Overall, caregiver interventions had a modest but significant benefit for caregiver knowledge, psychological morbidity, coping skills, and social support. Interventions did not appear to influence caregiver burden. A social skills training program showed a significant effect delay of nursing home admission and overall, 68% of interventions met the criteria for study success.	Heterogeneity of sample characteristics and study design and studies with small sample sizes are limitations.	Caregiver interventions have the potential to benefit patients and caregivers. Programs that involve the patients and their families and are more intensive and modified to caregivers' needs tend to be more successful.

Brodaty, H., Green, A., & Koschera, A. (2003). Meta-analysis of psychosocial interventions for caregivers of people with dementia. *Journal of the American Geriatrics Society, 51,* 657–664.

| Burns, Nichols, Martindale-Adams, Graney, & Lummus, 2003 | This study developed and tested two 24-mo primary care interventions to alleviate the psychological distress suffered by the caregivers of those with AD. | Level I RCT 167 caregiver-care recipient dyads | Intervention Interventions, using educational materials, were patient behavior management alone and patient behavior management plus caregiver stress-coping management. Outcome Measures ■ Health Status Scale ■ Modified General Well-Being Scale ■ Center for Epidemiologic Studies Depression Scale ■ RMBPC | During 24 mo, caregivers who received the patient behavior management component only, compared with those who also received the stress-coping component, had significantly worse outcomes for general well-being and a trend toward increased risk of depression. | The intervention contact time was shorter than planned for both groups because of unexpected intervening factors (i.e., scheduling conflicts). Sample size was too small to provide sufficient power to document statistical significance of interventions, although interventions appeared to be effective. | Brief care interventions may be effective in reducing caregiver distress and burden in the long-term management of the dementia patient. Interventions that focus only on care recipient behavior, without addressing caregiving issues, may not be as adequate for reducing caregiver distress. This type of intervention can also be useful given the chronic, progressive nature of dementia because it provides support to caregivers and assists them in differentiating progression of disease from their own limited skills. |

Burns, R., Nichols, L. O., Martindale-Adams, J., Graney, M. J., & Lummus, A. (2003). Primary care interventions for dementia caregivers: 2-year outcomes from the REACH study. *Gerontologist, 43,* 547–555.

(continued)

EVIDENCE TABLE: What is the effectiveness of educational and supportive strategies for caregivers of persons with dementia on the ability to maintain participation in that role? *(Contexts) (continued)*

Author/Year	Study Objectives	Level/Design/ Participants	Intervention and Outcome Measures	Results	Study Limitations	Implications for Occupational Therapy
Cooke, McNally, Mulligan, Harrison, & Newman, 2001	The objective was to identify the type of components (e.g. education, counseling) that have been used in psychosocial/ psychoeducational interventions for dementia caregivers, and to evaluate the success of the different components or combination of components in producing positive outcomes for dementia caregivers.	Level I Systematic review 40 studies	Intervention Interventions included improving the caregivers' psychological well-being or social well-being directly. Interventions included general education, general discussion, support group, social skills training, social support, social activities, cognitive problem solving, cognitive therapy, cognitive skills, practical caregiving skills, record keeping, relaxation, behavior therapy, psychotherapy and counseling, respite, and miscellaneous. Outcome Measures ■ AD Knowledge Test ■ Beck Depression Inventory ■ GHQ ■ Brief Symptom Inventory ■ Revised Memory Behavior Problem Checklist ■ Zarit Burden Inventory ■ Norbeck's Social Support Questionnaire ■ Instrumental and Expressive Social Support Scale ■ Negative Impact on Elderly-Caregiver Family Relationship Scale ■ Social Support Appraisals Scale	Overall, there is little evidence that interventions consistently produced benefits for caregivers in terms of improved caregiver psychological well-being, caregiver burden or social outcomes. However, these interventions rarely produced any deterioration in the outcomes measured. 1 study found that a group receiving telephone lectures showed improved levels of emotional support and knowledge about dementia when compared to a peer telephone network group. Interventions with social components were the most likely to show improvements on measures of psychological well-being rather than on burden. Caregiver interventions may require delay before their effects become apparent.	There was significantly varied sample size in studies (5–5,307) and high attrition rates (up to 64%) for long-term follow-up. Baseline levels of depression varied among studies. Caregiver burden measures appear insensitive to change.	It is possible to produce consistent improvement in caregivers' knowledge of the care recipient's illness, but knowledge appears unrelated to psychological and social outcomes. The inclusion of social and cognitive components appears to be relatively effective in improving psychological well-being.

Cooke, D. D., McNally, L., Mulligan, K. T., Harrison, M. J., & Newman, S. P. (2001). Psychosocial interventions for caregivers of people with dementia: A systematic review. *Aging and Mental Health, 5,* 120–135.

| Curry, Walker, & Hogstel, 2006 | The objective was to evaluate a pilot (Phase II) workplace educational project that addressed the most salient needs of employed caregivers. | Level III
1 group, nonrandomized, posttest

Participants
35 employees attended 1 or more sessions | Intervention
On the basis of a needs assessment completed by employees of a large institution, educational sessions were offered during 3 consecutive months.

3.5-hr educational sessions were offered during 3 consecutive months. Topics included specific health information, community resources, supplemental services, housing and long-term care options, Medicare/Medigap/other insurance, support groups, and end-of-life legal information.

Outcome Measures
Sessions were evaluated by participants on a 5-point Likert-type scale for usefulness of information, quality of presentation, and value of session. | Attendees found information valuable (relevant) to their caregiving responsibilities and useful in their caregiver role.

The 3 highest ranked content topics by value to attendees were normal aging vs. disease, Area Agency on Aging respite voucher information, and practical ideas/legal forms. | No baseline of knowledge was obtained for comparison. Sample size was small. Only 29% participated in all sessions. No statistical adjustments were made for inconsistencies in attendance. | Informational sessions are useful to increase caregiver knowledge and confidence in their roles. Caregivers particularly can use information about progression of disease, referral to community resources and practical ideas for caregiving, all of which should be part of a basic occupational therapy plan for people with AD dementia and their caregivers. |

Curry, L. C., Walker, C., & Hogstel, M. O. (2006). Educational needs of employed family caregivers of older adults: Evaluation of a workplace project. *Geriatric Nursing, 27*, 166–173.

(continued)

EVIDENCE TABLE: What is the effectiveness of educational and supportive strategies for caregivers of persons with dementia on the ability to maintain participation in that role? (Contexts) (continued)

Author/Year	Study Objectives	Level/Design/ Participants	Intervention and Outcome Measures	Results	Study Limitations	Implications for Occupational Therapy
Gitlin, Hauck, Dennis, & Winter, 2005	The objective was to examine whether treatment effects found at 6 mo after active treatment were sustained at 12 mo for family caregivers who participated in an occupational therapy intervention tested as part of the National Institutes of Health REACH initiative.	Level I Randomized Stratified 2-group design with 3 assessment points (baseline, 6 mo, and 12 mo) Participants Participants were 127 family caregivers who lived with a person who had dementia. All were age > 21, had been caregivers for > 6 mo, and provided > 4 hr of daily care to people with 1 or more activity limitations. 78.7% women 64.6% nonspouses 37% White 61% African-American 2% "other"	Intervention The experimental group received 6 occupational therapy sessions (five 90-min home visits and one telephone session) to help the family modify the environment to support daily function of the person with dementia and reduce caregiver burden. After 6-mo active treatment, a maintenance phase consisted of 1 home and 3 brief telephone sessions to reinforce strategy use and obtain closure. Occupational therapy sessions provided caregivers with education, problem-solving and technical skills (task-simplification, communication), and simple home modifications. Control group received the usual care. Outcome Measures ▪ REACH modified Revised Memory and Problem Behavior Checklist ▪ Single REACH vigilance item ▪ Days receiving ADLs help ▪ Task Management Strategy Index	At 6 mo, caregivers in intervention reported improved skills, less need for providing assistance, and fewer behavioral occurrences compared to the control group. At 12 mo, caregiver affect improved.	"Usual" care was not described for comparison. The sample size was small. Brief maintenance phase may not be sufficiently intensive to maintain gains in more domains	An in-home skills training program helps sustain caregiver affect; longer and more frequent professional contact and ongoing skills training may be necessary to maintain other clinically important outcomes such as reduced upset with behaviors.

Gitlin, L. N., Hauck, W. W., Dennis, M. P., & Winter, L. (2005). Maintenance of effects of the Home Environmental Skill-building Program for family caregivers and individuals with Alzheimer's disease and related disorders. *Journals of Gerontology. Series A, Biological Sciences and Medical Sciences, 60*, 368–374.

Author/Year	Study Objectives	Level/Design/Participants	Intervention and Outcome Measures	Results	Study Limitations	Implications for Occupational Therapy
Gitlin, Winter, Burke, Chernett, Dennis, & Hauck, 2008	The objective was to test whether the TAP reduces dementia-related neuropsychiatric behaviors, promotes activity engagement, and enhances caregiver well-being.	<u>Level I</u> RCT <u>Participants</u> 60 dementia patients and family caregivers. Dementia patients were English speaking, physician diagnosis or MMSE score < 24, able to feed self and participate in > 2 self-care activities. They were also primarily men (57%) and White (77%), with a mean age of 79. Caregivers were English-speaking, age ≥ 21, lived with the patient, and provided ≥ 4 hr of daily care.	<u>Intervention</u> Intervention consisted of six 90-min home visits and two 15-min telephone contacts. Home sessions of occupational therapy intervention involved neuropsychological and functional testing, selection and customization of activities to match capabilities identified in testing, and instruction to caregivers in use of activities. Main trial end-point was 4 mo. At 4 mo, control participants received the TAP intervention and were reassessed 4 mo later. <u>Outcome Measures</u> *Dementia Patient Outcomes:* ▪ Agitated Behaviors in Dementia Scale ▪ Revised Memory and Behavior Problem Checklist ▪ Cornell Scale for Depression in Dementia, Investigator-developed index of caregiver report of patient ▪ QoL–AD *Caregiver Outcomes:* ▪ Investigator-developed mastery scale, ▪ Zarit Burden Scale ▪ Objective burden estimated by caregiver ▪ CES-D	At 4 mo, compared with controls, intervention caregivers reported reduced frequency of problem behaviors (specifically for shadowing and repetitive questioning) and greater activity engagement, including the ability to keep busy. Fewer caregivers reported argumentation and agitation on the part of the patient. Caregiver benefits included fewer hours doing things and being on duty, greater mastery, self-efficacy, and skill enhancement. However, subjective appraisals of burden were not affected.	The study lacked an attention control group. There was reliance on caregiver self-report of behavioral occurrences, which may be affected by caregiver mood or perceived study demands.	Enhancements to patient function are likely to reduce the objective burden of caregivers, as measured by time spent on caregiving. However, interventions must also be designed to target caregivers' subjective well-being to complement patient intervention. Occupational therapy personnel should design interventions from which caregivers can derive or see immediate results. Further, enhanced understanding of preserved strengths of the patient as well as how to adapt activities to capitalize on those enhanced strengths are helpful for caregivers' sense of mastery and success in their role.

(continued)

EVIDENCE TABLE: What is the effectiveness of educational and supportive strategies for caregivers of persons with dementia on the ability to maintain participation in that role? (Contexts) (continued)

Author/Year	Study Objectives	Level/Design/ Participants	Intervention and Outcome Measures	Results	Study Limitations	Implications for Occupational Therapy
Gitlin, Winter, Burke, Chernett, Dennis, & Hauck, 2008 *(cont.)*			▪ Investigator-developed confidence using activities scale ▪ Task Management Strategy Index			

Gitlin, L., Winter, L., Burke, J., Chernett, N., Dennis, M., & Hauck, W. (2008). Tailored activities to manage neuropsychiatric behaviors in persons with dementia and reduce caregiver burden: A randomized pilot study. *American Journal of Geriatric Psychiatry, 16*, 229–239.

Graff, Adang, Vernooij-Dassen, Dekker, Jomsson, Thijssen, et al., 2008	The objective was to assess the cost effectiveness of community-based occupational therapy compared with usual care in older patients with dementia and their caregivers from a societal point.	<u>Level I</u> RCT <u>Participants</u> 135 patients aged ≥ 65 with mild to moderate dementia living in the community and their primary caregivers	<u>Intervention</u> Intervention consisted of 10 1-hr sessions of occupational therapy held over 5 wk, including cognitive and behavioral interventions, to train patients in the use of aids to compensate for cognitive decline and caregivers in coping behaviors and supervision. Treatment delivered by experienced occupational therapists included 4 sessions of diagnostics and goal defining for patients and caregivers to choose meaningful activities. Environmental modifications and compensatory strategies were used to adapt activities of daily living. In the remaining 6 sessions, patients were taught to optimize compensatory and environmental strategies to improve ADL performance. Primary caregivers were trained by means of cognitive and behavioral interventions to use effective supervision, problem solving, and coping strategies	The economic evaluation showed an average savings of $2,621 per couple successfully treated with occupational therapy. The probability of occupational therapy being the dominant and most efficient intervention was estimated to be 94%.	Lack of inclusion of a generic quality-of-life measure limits comparability with other interventions. It is not possible to carry out a double-blind study. This was a nonrepresentative, convenience sample.	Occupational therapy professionals are best equipped to carry out the specific tasks of this intervention. Community occupational therapy is a highly effective, cost-effective therapy for community-dwelling elders and their caregivers and should be advocated as an included service in all community health services, primary care services, and outpatient services for people with dementia.

to sustain the patient's and their own autonomy and social participation.

Control group received no occupational therapy during the study period but did receive occupational therapy 12 wk after the completion of the study.

Outcome Measures
Primary outcome measure for patient function was process scale of AMPS.

Primary outcome for caregivers was assessed with the Sense of Competence Questionnaire.

Over 3 mo, primary outcomes were combined in 1 measure for successful treatment for economic evaluation. Cost analysis measures included caregivers' records of patients' visits to the general practitioner, physiotherapist, social worker, or other health care suppliers specifically related to dementia. Caregivers also recorded their own visits to health care services and hours spent in care of the patient. Number of hours patient received treatment at home as well as if they received meals on wheels was tracked.

Graff, M., Adang, E., Vernooji-Dassen, M., Dekker, J., Jomsson, L, Thijssen, M., et al. (2008). Community occupational therapy for older patients with dementia and their care givers: Cost effectiveness study. *British Medical Journal, 336,* 134–138.

(continued)

Caregiver

EVIDENCE TABLE: What is the effectiveness of educational and supportive strategies for caregivers of persons with dementia on the ability to maintain participation in that role? *(Contexts) (continued)*

Author/Year	Study Objectives	Level/Design/ Participants	Intervention and Outcome Measures	Results	Study Limitations	Implications for Occupational Therapy
Graff, Vernooij-Dassen, Thijssen, Dekker, Hoefnagels, & Rikkert, 2006	The objective was to determine the effectiveness of community-based occupational therapy on daily functioning of patients with dementia and the sense of competence of their caregivers.	<u>Level I</u> RCT <u>Participants</u> 135 patients age ≥ 65 with mild to moderate dementia living in the community and their primary caregivers	<u>Intervention</u> Intervention consisted of 1-hr sessions of occupational therapy held over 5 wk, including cognitive and behavioral interventions, to train patients in the use of aids to compensate for cognitive decline and caregivers in coping behaviors and supervision. Treatment delivered by experienced occupational therapists included 4 sessions of diagnostics and goal defining for patients and caregivers to choose meaningful activities. Environmental modifications and compensatory strategies were used to adapt activities of daily living. In the remaining 6 sessions, patients were taught to optimize compensatory and environmental strategies to improve ADLs performance. Control group received occupational therapy 12 wk after the completion of the study. <u>Outcome Measures</u> *Patient:* ■ MMSE ■ BCRS ■ GDS ■ Revised Memory and Behavioral Problems Checklist	At 6 wk there were significant differences between treatment and control groups. Patients who received occupational therapy functioned significantly better in daily life than those in the control group. Primary caregivers who received occupational therapy felt significantly more competent than those who did not. Statistical analysis showed significant differences in scores for patient and caregiver groups. At 12 wk, differences between patient and caregiver groups remained significant, and 75% of patients in the intervention group had clinically relevant improvement from the 6th week assessment compared with 9% of the control group.	Authors were not able to carry out double-blind study conditions. This was an unrepresentative sample, recruited from 1 university hospital. The study lacked an attention control group.	10 sessions of community occupational therapy given over 5 wk improved the daily functioning of patients with dementia and diminished the burden on caregivers. Benefits to the patient appear to be sustained when caregivers are trained to provide supervision to patients and when they are provided with individual support.

Graff, Vernooij-Dassen, Thijssen, Dekker, Hoefnagels, & Rikkert, 2006 *(conti.)*

- Process Scale of the AMPS
- Age, sex, and educational level
- comorbidity

Caregivers:
- Sense of Competence Questionnaire
- Center for Epidemiologic Studies Depression Scale

Graff, M. J. L., Vernooij-Dassen, M. J. M., Thijssen, M., Dekker, J., Hoefnagels, W. H. L., & Rikkert, M. G. M. (2006). Community-based occupational therapy for patients with dementia and their caregivers: Randomized controlled trial. *British Medical Journal, 333,* 1196–1201.

| Graff, Vernooij-Dassen, Thijssen, Dekker, Hoefnagels, & Rikkert, 2007 | The objective was to investigate the effects of community occupational therapy on dementia patients' and caregivers' quality of life, mood, and health status and caregivers' sense of control over life. | <u>Level I</u>
RCT

<u>Participants</u>
135 patients aged ≥ 65 with mild to moderate dementia living in the community and their primary caregivers | <u>Intervention</u>
Intervention consisted of 10 1-hour sessions of occupational therapy held over 5 wk, including cognitive and behavioral interventions, to train patients in the use of aids to compensate for cognitive decline and caregivers in coping behaviors and supervision. Treatment delivered by experienced occupational therapists included 4 sessions of diagnostics and goal defining for patients and caregivers to choose meaningful activities. Environmental modifications and compensatory strategies were used to adapt activities of daily living. In the remaining 6 sessions, patients were taught to optimize compensatory and environmental strategies to improve ADLs performance. | All overall scores at 6 wk differed significantly between the intervention and control group. Patients and informal caregivers who received occupational therapy improved significantly relative to baseline as compared to controls on overall quality of life, health status, and patient and caregiver mood.

At 12 wk, all significant outcomes remained significant for the intervention group as compared to control. | It was not possible to carry out a double-blind study. This was a nonrepresentative, convenience sample. | This study suggests that there is a strong positive association between dementia patients' daily functioning, mood, and quality of life on caregivers' sense of control over life. Training caregivers in supervision skills and providing them with individualized support as part of the occupational therapy plan for patients with dementia is an essential component of occupational therapy treatment for this population. |

(continued)

EVIDENCE TABLE: What is the effectiveness of educational and supportive strategies for caregivers of persons with dementia on the ability to maintain participation in that role? (Contexts) (continued)

Author/Year	Study Objectives	Level/Design/ Participants	Intervention and Outcome Measures	Results	Study Limitations	Implications for Occupational Therapy
Graff, Vernooij-Dassen, Thijssen, Dekker, Hoefnagels, & Rikkert, 2007 (cont.)			Primary caregivers were trained by means of cognitive and behavioral interventions to use effective supervision, problem-solving, and coping strategies to sustain the patient's and their own autonomy and social participation. Control group received no occupational therapy during the study period, but did receive occupational therapy 12 wk after the completion of the study. Outcome Measures ■ Occupational Performance History Interview ■ COPM ■ Ethnographic interview ■ Dementia Quality of Life Instrument ■ GHQ ■ Cornell Scale for Depression ■ Center for Epidemiologic Studies Depression Scale ■ Mastery Scale ■ Cumulative Illness Rating Scale for Geriatrics ■ MMSE ■ Revised Memory and Behavioral Problems Checklist ■ Caregiver relationship with the patient			

Graff, M., Vernooij-Dassen, M., Thijssen, M., Deller, J., Hoefnagels, W., & Rikkert, M. (2007). Effects of community occupational therapy on quality of life, mood, and health status in dementia patients and their caregivers: A randomized controlled trial. *Journal of Gerontology: Medical Sciences, 62A*, 1002–1009.

Hepburn, Lewis, Narayan, Center, Tornatore, Bremer, et al., 2005	The objective was to test the ability of a psychoeducational intervention to relieve or forestall dementia caregiver distress over a 1-yr period.	Level I RCT Participants 215 self-selected care giver/care receiver dyads recruited from a variety of community sources over a 2-yr period	Intervention Partners in Caregiving program consisted of 2 versions of a multisession multidisciplinary program: *Experimental group #1:* Program concentrated on development of strategies for day-to-day caregiving. *Experimental group #2:* Program consisted of caregiving practice in a de-cision-making framework, identifying and using values and preferences as a way to evaluate the options available in day-to-day caregiving decisions. Each program met for 2 hr/wk over a period of 6 wk. Programs were led by teams of study investigators (2 leaders per group). *Control Group:* Wait list controls <u>Outcome Measures</u> ▪ MMSE (care-recipient) ▪ Open-Ended Interview ▪ Questionnaire (developed for study) that included scales reporting care recipients' abilities and caregiver perceptions ▪ Follow-up telephone in-terview at 6 and 12 mo ▪ Caregiver Distress Measure	The trial initially was designed to compare the effectiveness of both experimental interventions, but preliminary examina-tion revealed no important differences in effect. Thus, the data from the 2 intervention groups were combined for comparison with controls. Strengthening caregivers' ability to better under-stand and undertake their caregiving role staves off increasing distress and improves caregiving at-titude at 6 mo. However, at 1 yr, between-group effects deteriorated, although still indicated persistence of effect.	This was a convenience sample; all measures were self-reported.	Given the progressive nature of dementing disorders, a reasonable goal of caregiver interven-tion for occupational therapy professionals is the maintenance (rather than improvement) of caregiver well-being. This study suggests that in addition to the traditional focus on caregiving skills occupational therapy personnel are likely to offer, additional focus should be placed on care-givers' appraisal of their situation and skills.

Hepburn, K., Lewis, M., Narayan, S., Center, B., Tornatore, J., Bremer, K., et al. (2005). Partners in caregiving: A psychoeducation program affecting dementia family caregivers' distress and caregiving outlook. *Clinical Gerontologist 29,* 53–69.

(continued)

Caregiver

EVIDENCE TABLE: What is the effectiveness of educational and supportive strategies for caregivers of persons with dementia on the ability to maintain participation in that role? (Contexts) (continued)

Author/Year	Study Objectives	Level/Design/ Participants	Intervention and Outcome Measures	Results	Study Limitations	Implications for Occupational Therapy
Hepburn, Tornatore, Center, & Ostwald, 2001	The objective was to test a role-training intervention as a way to help family caregivers appreciate and assume a more clinical belief set about caregiving and thereby ameliorate the adverse outcomes associated with caregiving.	<u>Level I</u> RCT <u>Participants</u> 117 caregiver–care receiver dyads referred from a wide variety of community agencies. Care receivers were mostly men (55.6%) with a mean age of 77. Severity of dementia had not progressed beyond the Functional Assessment Staging 7b stage. Caregivers were mostly women (70%) with a mean age of 65. Caregivers were spouses (65.5%) and children (28.3%) of care receivers. All participants identified themselves as White.	<u>Intervention</u> Family care receiver dyads were randomly assigned to training beginning immediately or were placed in a waitlist control group and assigned to receive training in 5 to 6 mo, after completion of data collection. Treatment: 2 hrs/session over 7 wk was provided using a program based on a stress and coping theory framework. The curriculum combined classroom instruction and exercises and assignments to read additional materials. The training included 5 main components: ■ Information provision ■ Concept development ■ Role clarification ■ Belief clarification ■ Mastery-focused coaching Training was provided in group settings in weekly 2-hr sessions over the course of 7 wk. Workshop faculty was made up of a multidisciplinary team (nurse, educator, family therapist, occupational therapist). While caregivers and other family members attended the training, a day care-like group was provided for care receivers.	Significant within-group improvements occurred 3 mo after intervention with treatment group caregivers on measures of beliefs about caregiving and reaction to behavior. When outcomes were compared, treatment group caregivers were significantly different (in the expected direction) from those in the control group on measures of the stress mediator, beliefs, key outcomes, response to behavior, depression, and burden. There was a significant positive association between the strengthened mediator, the caregivers' having less emotionally enmeshed beliefs about caregiving roles and responsibilities, and the outcome, namely improvements in burden ($p = .019$) and depression ($p = .007$).	The following concerns were limitations: ■ Homogeneous sample ■ Large attrition ■ Caregivers were help-seekers ■ Results only measured at 3 mo; long-term effects not measured ■ Caregiver knowledge changes not measured ■ Instrument (Beliefs About Caregiving Scale) not specifically validated for caregivers of people with dementia	Although the results of this study require careful interpretation because the type of dementia was not specified and the main tool used for outcome measurement was not validated for caregivers of people with dementia, there is evidence that caregivers appear to benefit from information provided in an ongoing manner, respond to specific information about available services (e.g., quality, reasonable expectation, length), and coaching (particularly to understand that the caregiving role is different from other family roles).

					Outcome Measures		
					■ MMSE ■ Lawton ADL Scale ■ Revised Memory and Behavior Problem Checklist ■ Beliefs About Caregiving Scale ■ Center for Epidemiologic Studies Depression Scale ■ Revised Zarit Burden Scale		

Hepburn, K. W., Tornatore, J., Center, B., & Ostwald, S. W. (2001). Dementia family caregiver training: Affecting beliefs about caregiving and caregiver outcomes. *Journal of the American Geriatrics Society, 49,* 450–457.

Author/Year	Objective	Level/Design	Participants	Intervention	Results	Implications
Hosaka & Sugiyama, 2003	The objective was to investigate the effects of a group structured intervention on the mental and physical discomfort and immune function of family caregivers of people with dementia in Japan.	Level III 1 group Pre–post assessment Participants 20 women family caregivers Median age 54.7 (range 47–66) Period of home care ranged from 1–12 yr (mean 5.8) 8 care recipients had AD dementia, and 10 had vascular dementia.	Intervention 5 wk structured group intervention consisted of one 90-min session/wk. Participants listened to lectures provided by the researchers; participated in progressive muscle relaxation exercises using a 15-min audiotape produced for this study; and participated in group discussion. Outcome Measures ■ Profile of Mood States ■ GHQ-30	Significant improvement (*p* < .05) in the scores of depression, anger–hostility, fatigue, and confusion, physical symptoms, anxiety–mood disorder, and suicidality–depression.	Sample was a convenience sample and small. This study suggests occupational therapy professionals should include discussion and social support opportunities in caregiver training. In addition, assisting caregivers in developing basic relaxation skills through autogenic training aids can help improve their own well-being.

Hosaka, T., & Sugiyama, Y. (2003). Structured intervention in family caregivers of the demented elderly and changes in their immune function. *Psychiatry and Clinical Neurosciences, 57,* 147–151.

(continued)

EVIDENCE TABLE: What is the effectiveness of educational and supportive strategies for caregivers of persons with dementia on the ability to maintain participation in that role? *(Contexts) (continued)*

Author/Year	Study Objectives	Level/Design/ Participants	Intervention and Outcome Measures	Results	Study Limitations	Implications for Occupational Therapy
Huang, Lotus Shyu, Chen, Chen, & Lin, 2003	The objective was to investigate the effectiveness of a home-based caregiver training program for caregivers of elders with dementia and behavioral problems in Taiwan.	Level I RCT Participants 48 patients with dementia and their caregivers	Intervention Experimental group (n = 24) received 2 in-home caregiving training sessions (separated by 1 wk) provided by 1 of the investigators. The initial visit focused on obtaining assessment data on the conditions of the dementia patient, identification of targeted behavioral problems, and exploration of the causative environmental stimuli. The second visit further assessed family resources and finalized the plan for handling specific behavior problems with the caregiver. 2 telephone consultations focused on targeted behaviors. The training program was based on the Progressively Lowered Stress Threshold model. Control group received educational materials and 2 social telephone calls (every 2 wk). Outcome Measures ■ Chinese version of the CMAI (for care recipient) ■ Agitation Management Self-Efficacy Scale (for caregiver) Measures obtained at baseline, 3 wk, and 3 mo after intervention.	The care-recipient scores of physically nonaggressive behavior, verbally aggressive, and nonaggressive subscales decreased significantly and continuously. Caregivers' scores on the Agitation Management Self-Efficacy Scale increased significantly and continuously in the experimental group.	Small sample, convenience sample, and short follow-up may not indicate true effect of intervention.	Caregiver training, even of short duration, can help both decrease non–physically aggressive behavioral symptoms of care recipients with dementia and increase the sense of self-efficacy of caregivers. Occupational therapy professionals should take care of helping caregivers understand the progressive nature of the disease as well as causative environmental factors associated with behavioral problems. Collaboration with the caregiver in targeting problems is more likely to result in greater sense of self-efficacy than when only following prescribed interventions.

Huang, H. L., Lotus Shyu, Y. I., Chen, M. C., Chen, S. T., & Lin, L. C. (2003). A pilot study on a home-based caregiver training program for improving caregiver self-efficacy and decreasing the behavioral problems of elders with dementia in Taiwan. *International Journal of Geriatric Psychiatry, 18*(4), 337–345.

| Kuhn & Mendes de Leon, 2001 | The objective was to investigate the effectiveness of an AD dementia knowledge-building program in increasing caregiver knowledge of the disease and their management of their feelings about early AD-related problems and emotions as well as reduce their depression. | Level III
1 group
Pretest–posttest

Participants
58 caregivers of 38 patients
Caregivers were 74% women, average age 54

Participants recruited from 2 outpatient clinics and 2 continuing care retirement communities | Intervention
5 consecutive weekly sessions, each 2 hr long. Psychoeducational model focused on the medical, psychological, and social issues associated with the early stages of AD. Format of each session included lecture, slides, and discussion reinforced by the training manual.

Outcome Measures
(pre, post, and 9 mo follow-up)
■ AD Knowledge Test
■ RMBPC
■ CES-D
■ Brief survey completed at end of intervention asking participants to evaluate helpfulness of program | Significant improvement was reported in AD knowledge (effect size of 0.8). There were no statistically significant changes in caregiver reports on the RMBPC or CES-D noted.

At 9 mo posttest, AD knowledge remained intact, and no significant changes were noted on the RMBPC or CES-D. | Study lacked control group. Sample was a convenience sample and relatively homogeneous. | Psychoeducation is effective in increasing the knowledge of caregivers related to the progression of the disease and its symptoms. Knowledge of AD does not necessarily translate into decreased burden or less depression on the part of caregivers. Occupational therapy professionals should certainly educate caregivers about the disease in addition to finding other forms of intervention for support in order to assist caregivers in remaining in that role and having a sense of success and mastery. |

Kuhn, D. R., & Mendes de León, C. F. (2001). Evaluating an educational intervention with relatives of persons in the early stages of Alzheimer's disease. *Research on Social Work Practice, 11,* 531–548.

(continued)

EVIDENCE TABLE: What is the effectiveness of educational and supportive strategies for caregivers of persons with dementia on the ability to maintain participation in that role? (Contexts) (continued)

Author/Year	Study Objectives	Level/Design/ Participants	Intervention and Outcome Measures	Results	Study Limitations	Implications for Occupational Therapy
Lee & Cameron, 2004	The objective was to assess the effects of respite care for people with dementia and their caregivers, in particular the effect of respite care on rates of institutionalization.	<u>Level I</u> Systematic review 3 RCTs were included in this review.	<u>Intervention</u> Review included studies providing interventions aimed to provide rest or respite for the primary caregiver. <u>Outcome Measures</u> • Brief Symptom Inventory–Global Severity Index • Mortality • Number of days living in the community • CES-D • Bradburn Affect Balance Scale • Zarit's Caregiver Burden Scale • Duke–UC Functional Support Questionnaire • Health and Social Service Utilization	Current evidence does not demonstrate any benefits or adverse effects from the use of respite care for people with dementia or their caregivers.	Small number (3) of studies met criteria for inclusion.	Results should be treated with caution because they may reflect the lack of high quality research in the area rather than lack of benefit.

Lee, H., & Cameron, M. (2004). Respite care for people with dementia and their carers. *Cochrane Database of Systematic Reviews*, Issue 1. Art. No.: CD004396. doi: 10.1002/14651858. CD004396. pub2

Author/Year	Study Objectives	Level/Design/ Participants	Intervention and Outcome Measures	Results	Study Limitations	Implications for Occupational Therapy
Mahoney, Tarlow, Jones, Tennstedt, & Kasten, 2001	The objective was to investigate the usefulness of a computer-mediated interactive voice response system integrated with voice-mail to help family caregivers manage disruptive behaviors in people with AD.	<u>Level I</u> RCT. <u>Participants</u> 100 caregivers who were age > 21 and provided ≥ 4 hr per day of assistance or supervision for a minimum of 6 mo	<u>Intervention</u> Intervention group received training on how to use the REACH Telephone Linked Care. This system provided access to 4 intervention modules: • Monitoring and counsel-ing (provided weekly)	Usage fell over the first 4 mo and reached a pla-teau beyond the 4th mo. Adopters were significantly older, more highly educated, and reported a greater sense of manage-ment of the situation than nonadopters. The majority	Small sample extent	Occupational therapy pro-fessionals can participate in the development of such a service, particularly following direct provision of service. A particular role for occupational therapy personnel could be in providing advice and monitoring progress. Low

Participants came from 60 recruitment sites.

- In-home support group (voicemail system designed to mimic a computer chat group).
- Ask-the-expert (confidential voicemail) access to a multidisciplinary AD expert panel
- Activity/caregiver respite conversation (18 min automated interactive voice response telephone conversation using a soothing, didactic manner for the person with AD).

System was available to intervention group for 12 mo.

Control group received usual care and were offered the Telephone Linked Care system at the conclusion of the study period.

Outcome Measures
- Technology: Use of technology
- Proficiency: Level of skill using the Telephone Linked Care
- User characteristics (e.g., gender, age)
- Perceived stress
- Mastery: 7-point scale of sense of control
- Management of situation: Indication of caregiver coping measured on a 3-point index
- Care recipient characteristics: Measure using the MMSE, dependencies in ADLs, and IADLs scales

of participants reported that using the Telephone Linked Care was not difficult.

The weekly caregiver conversation, providing monitoring and advice, was the most frequently used module of the 4. The respite call module was the second most frequently used. The ask-the-expert and bulletin board modules were the least used.

Most participants preferred in-person support meetings, and were clear about the importance of human contact for them.

tolerance for technological difficulties should be considered, and the importance person-to-person contact should be considered in setting up this type of program.

Mahoney, D. M., Tarlow, B., Jones, R. N., Tennstedt, S., & Kasten, L. (2001). Factors affecting the use of a telephone-based intervention for caregivers of people with Alzheimer's disease. *Journal of Telemedicine and Telecare, 7,* 139–148.

(continued)

Caregiver

EVIDENCE TABLE: What is the effectiveness of educational and supportive strategies for caregivers of persons with dementia on the ability to maintain participation in that role? (Contexts) (continued)

Author/Year	Study Objectives	Level/Design/ Participants	Intervention and Outcome Measures	Results	Study Limitations	Implications for Occupational Therapy
Mittelman, Ferris, Shulman, Steingberg, & Levin, 1996	The objective was to determine the long-term effectiveness of comprehensive support and counseling for spouse-caregivers and families in postponing or preventing nursing home placement of patients with AD.	<u>Level I</u> RCT <u>Participants</u> 206 spouse-caregivers of AD patients recruited over a 3½ yr period from community clinics and centers in New York City (58.3% women)	<u>Intervention</u> Treatment consisted of the following components: ■ 2 individual and 4 family counseling sessions in the first 4 mo after caregiver enrolled in the study; sessions were task-oriented and focused on communication, problem solving, and improving emotional and instrumental support of primary caregiver. ■ Weekly support group for caregivers after initial 4 mo of participation in study. ■ Continuous availability of counselors to caregivers and families to help deal with the changing nature and severity of the patient's symptoms. ■ Access to counseling on an ongoing basis. The control group received usual care. <u>Outcome Measures</u> ■ GDS ■ Memory and Behavior Problem Checklist ■ Social Network Questionnaire	Both caregiver depression and reaction to troublesome behavior were significant predictors of placement. Median time from baseline to nursing home placement was 329 days longer for the treatment group than the control group.	Support group participation was required of caregivers in the treatment group but not denied to caregivers in control group. 72% of caregivers in the treatment group and 40.8% in the control group joined a support group, so results related to support group not unique to tested intervention.	Occupational therapy professionals can be part of a team providing support and information to spouse-caregivers. Information about progression of disease, personal coping skills, and management strategies is particularly useful. Occupational therapy professionals should monitor caregiver depression and provide resources for support groups for caregivers. Such interventions are likely to result in delayed nursing home placement.

Mittelman, M. S., Ferris, S. H., Shulman, E., Steingberg, G., & Levin, B. (1996). A family intervention to delay nursing home placement of patients with Alzheimer's disease: A randomized controlled trial. *Journal of the American Medical Association, 276*, 1725–1731.

Author/Year	Study Objectives	Level/Design/Participants	Intervention and Outcome Measures	Results	Study Limitations/Implications
Mittelman, Haley, Clay, & Roth, 2006	The objective was to determine the effectiveness of a counseling and support intervention for spouse-caregivers in delaying time to nursing home placement of patients with AD and to identify the mechanisms through which the intervention accomplished this goal.	Level I RCT As above. Participants 406 spouse-caregivers of AD patients recruited over a 8½ yr period from community clinics and centers in New York City 60.1% women 90.9% White 75.8% of care receivers had mild to moderate dementia at baseline Caregivers followed longitudinally for up to 17 yr	Intervention As above. All caregivers were interviewed at regular intervals after entry into the study every 4 mo during the first year, and every 6 mo thereafter. Treatment group participants received counseling (2 individual and 4 family sessions), participated in support groups, and received ad-hoc telephone support/counseling. Control group participants were provided with normal counseling services offered to all families of the NYU Aging and Dementia Research Center. Outcome Measures ■ Memory and Behavior Problem Checklist ■ 3 questions from the physical health section of the Alder Americans Resources and Services questionnaire ■ Social Ne2rk Questionnaire ■ GDS	Caregivers in the intervention group were able to keep their spouses at home longer than caregivers in the usual care group. Higher patient income was predictive of longer time to placement. Increased severity of dementia, poorer caregiver physical health, lower satisfaction with social support, greater frequency of memory and behavior problems, more symptoms of depression, and higher caregiver burden were all significant predictors of higher nursing home placement rates.	As above, homogeneous sample relative to race (> 90% White) was a concern. Support group participation was required of caregivers in the treatment group but not denied to caregivers in the control group, so results related to support group were not unique to tested intervention. Despite use of random assignment, there were imbalances at baseline between treatment and control groups on several measures. Stratification may solve this problem in the future. Occupational therapy professionals should be alert to circumstances in which placement should be recommended to protect the caregivers' health and well-being.

Mittelman, M. S., Haley, W. E., Clay, O. J., & Roth, D. L. (2006). Improving caregiver well-being delays nursing home placement of patients with Alzheimer disease. *Neurology, 4*, 1592–1599.

Author/Year	Study Objectives	Level/Design/Participants	Intervention and Outcome Measures	Results	Study Limitations/Implications
Mittelman, Roth, Clay, & Haley, 2007	The objective was to determine the effects of counseling and educational support on the physical health of spouse caregivers of people with AD.	Level I RCT Participants 406 spouse caregivers of community-dwelling patients recruited	Intervention As above. 2 individual counseling sessions tailored to each caregiver's specific situation; 4 family	The control group reported significantly better subjective sense of health than the control group at 4 mo follow-up. The statistically significant difference between the 2 groups	As above, this was a relatively homogeneous sample. Participants in the control group received benefit from the	Psychosocial intervention for caregivers, emphasizing enhancement of social support, are likely to lead to improvements in caregiver health. Encouraging caregivers

(continued)

EVIDENCE TABLE: What is the effectiveness of educational and supportive strategies for caregivers of persons with dementia on the ability to maintain participation in that role? *(Contexts) (continued)*

Author/Year	Study Objectives	Level/Design/ Participants	Intervention and Outcome Measures	Results	Study Limitations	Implications for Occupational Therapy
Mittelman, Roth, Clay, & Haley, 2007 *(cont.)*		over a 9.5 yr period recruited through the NYU Alzheimer's Disease Center and referred from New York City's Chapter of the Alzheimer's association	counseling sessions with the primary caregiver and family members selected by the caregiver; encouragement and participation in locally available support groups that met weekly after the 4 mo follow-up; and continuous availability of counselors to caregivers and families by telephone (ad hoc counseling). Control group received usual care, but were given information on request. They did not receive individual or family counseling, nor were they asked to join a support group, although many did on their own. Outcome Measures ■ Questionnaire adapted from the OARS ■ GDS ■ Social Network Questionnaire	was maintained over the first 2 yr of follow-up. Depressive symptoms were a significant predictor of subjective sense of health. The findings suggest that enhanced support intervention led to a significant benefit to caregivers' self-rated health.	availability of counseling on an as-needed basis, which may have decreased the apparent differential effect of the intervention.	to strengthen their social support system should be a basic component of occupational therapy intervention for this population. Social support interventions should be structured and be provided over a long period of time.

Mittelman, M. S., Roth, D. L., Clay, O. J., & Haley, W. E. (2007). Preserving health of Alzheimer caregivers: Impact of a spouse caregiver intervention. *American Journal of Geriatric Psychiatry, 15,* 780–789.

| Mittelman, Roth, Haley, & Zarit, 2004 | The objective was to examine the effect of a caregiver program over a 4-yr period on both the frequency of problem behavior in people with AD and the reactions of their family caregivers. | Level I RCT

Participants
406 spouse-caregivers of AD patients recruited over a 8½ yr period from community clinics and centers in New York City

60.1% women
90.9% White
75.8% of care receivers had mild to moderate dementia at baseline

Caregivers followed longitudinally for up to 12 yr | Intervention
All caregivers were interviewed at regular intervals after entry into the study every 4 mo during the first yr, and every 6 mo thereafter.

Treatment group participants received counseling (2 individual and 4 family sessions) to focus on communication, problem solving, and education, depending on family needs. Also support groups and ad hoc telephone support/counseling were included.

The control group received usual care.

Outcome Measures
■ Memory and Behavior Problem Checklist
■ Social Network Questionnaire
■ GDS | Caregivers in the active treatment condition reported lower reaction scores (bother), on average, than usual care caregivers across all assessments after baseline. | This was a homogeneous sample relative to race (> 90% White). Support group participation was required of caregivers in the treatment group but not denied to caregivers in control group, so results related to support group not unique to tested intervention. | Psychosocial intervention that includes education and support and can provide caregivers with strategies to help them manage their reactions to behavior problems more effectively. This, in turn, can have a favorable effect on caregiver depression and nursing home placement. |

Mittelman, M. S., Roth, D. L., Haley, W. E., & Zarit, S. H. (2004). Effects of a caregiver intervention on negative caregiver appraisals of behavior problems in patients with Alzheimer's disease: Results of a randomized trial. *Journals of Gerontology, 59,* 27–34.

(continued)

EVIDENCE TABLE: What is the effectiveness of educational and supportive strategies for caregivers of persons with dementia on the ability to maintain participation in that role? (Contexts) (continued)

Author/Year	Study Objectives	Level/Design/ Participants	Intervention and Outcome Measures	Results	Study Limitations	Implications for Occupational Therapy
Peacock & Forbes, 2003	The objective was to assess the effectiveness of interventions designed to enhance the well-being of caregivers of people with dementia.	Level I Systematic review 36 studies (11 rated as "strong," 11 as "moderate," 13 as "weak," and 1 as "poor")	Intervention Studies reported on 4 types of intervention: education, case management, psychotherapy, and computer networking. Outcome Measures Most commonly measured outcome was institutionalization of the care recipient, followed by death of the care recipient, perceived behavior disturbances of the care recipient, caregiver depression, caregiver strain, stress, and use of formal services.	No 1 intervention had an overall significant impact on the well-being of caregivers. Case management did double the likelihood of intervention groups using community services, but did not affect levels of depression or strain of caregivers. Results indicated that education interventions are insufficient to improve overall caregiver psychological well-being; however, results indicated that institutionalization and death of the care recipient were delayed with caregiver training programs.	Most studies had methodological problems, such as not piloting tools or assessing appropriateness of tools for the population. Most studies recruited participants who already had accessed services, making it difficult to distinguish the degree to which results of trials were related to tested interventions.	Use of computers in networking interventions is especially interesting for rural caregivers and may increase in relevance as technology becomes more advanced. Case management was effective in increasing the use of formal services. Occupational therapy professionals should consider participating in such interventions and providing consultations and recommendations through computer networks.

Peacock, S. C., & Forbes, D. A. (2003). Interventions for caregivers of persons with dementia: A systematic review. *Canadian Journal of Nursing Research, 35,* 88–107.

Schacke & Zank, 2006	The objective was to evaluate the effectiveness of adult day care programs as supports for family caregivers of patients with dementia.	**Level II** Nonrandomized, controlled trial with qualitative, semistructured interview **Participants** 77 caregivers Average age = 58 87% women 41% employed 57% were caregiving children 32% were spouses Care recipients were on average 80 yr old, 73% were women, and on average already severely demented according to the MMSE. Participants recruited from an undetermined number of adult day care programs and through community centers.	**Intervention** Treatment group consisted of adult day care users. Day care offered group activities including cognitive stimulation, ADLs training, or gymnastics. The control group consisted of nonusers of adult day care. Both groups were interviewed for a baseline on initiation of the study and then again at 9 mo. The interview focused on 4 domains of caregiver stress: objective caregiving tasks, perceived stress caused by patient behavior problems, perceived restrictions concerning personal needs, and perceived role conflicts between care and family/job obligations. **Outcomes Measures** ▪ MMSE used to evaluate severity of dementia of care receivers ▪ Caregiving stress scale developed for present study	Use of day care is significantly effective in alleviating care-related stress, especially with regard to compatibility of family, job, and caregiving responsibilities. Further, it enhances caregivers' opportunity to take part in social and recreational activities. Adult day care programs were selectively effective in reducing stress associated with stereotyped patient behavior problems. Intervention did not appear to be effective in reducing caregiving tasks (i.e., supervision of the patient).	Differences between intervention and control group composition were not reported (i.e., length of time using adult day care). Sample size was small. Variability between programs offered at the adult day care center not accounted for. Attrition rate was high (48.6% of treatment group and 45% of control group). Baseline was obtained after patient and caregivers had become accustomed to the day care program, which may account for lack of change in certain measures between baseline and 9 mo follow-up interviews.	Occupational therapy professionals should encourage the use of adult day programs, recognizing that they alleviate some, but not all aspects of caregiving stress. Occupational therapy services can provide services not provided by adult day care programs, particularly in training caregivers on how to provide supervision for the patient. In addition, occupational therapy professionals should provide information regarding range of services available in the community.

Schacke, C., & Zank, S. R. (2006). Measuring the effectiveness of adult day care as a facility to support family caregivers of dementia patients. *Journal of Applied Gerontology, 25*(1), 65–81.

(continued)

EVIDENCE TABLE: What is the effectiveness of educational and supportive strategies for caregivers of persons with dementia on the ability to maintain participation in that role? (Contexts) (continued)

Author/Year	Study Objectives	Level/Design/ Participants	Intervention and Outcome Measures	Results	Study Limitations	Implications for Occupational Therapy
Schulz, R., O'Brien, A., Czaja, Ory, Norris, Martire, et. al., 2002	This article was a review of intervention studies that reported dementia caregiver outcomes published between 1996 and 2001, including psychosocial interventions for caregivers and environmental and pharmacological interventions for care recipients.	Level I Systematic review 52 reports on 43 distinct studies (27 used random assignment of participants to treatment conditions)	Intervention Interventions were design to achieve effects on caregiver *symptomatology* and included a variety of educational and psychotherapeutic interventions such as problem solving, coping skills training, behavior management, and support groups. Interventions designed to address caregiver *quality of life* included support groups, psychoeducational programs, stress management training, behavioral management, and environmentally focused occupational therapy. Interventions focused on *social significance* included residential care placement, patient longevity, and patient functional status. Outcome Measures Outcome measures were categorized according to 4 proposed areas of clinical significance: • Symptomatology • Quality of life • Social significance • Social validity	*Symptomatology:* There were small to modest improvements in depression symptoms for interventions in comparison to control conditions; benefits of interventions for anxiety appear to be equivocal; findings supporting a beneficial impact of intervention on distress are limited. *Quality of life:* Overall, these studies suggested that statistically significant reductions of burden, mood, and perceived stress can be achieved with some populations of caregivers, but the evidence of effect is mixed with regards to social support and marital satisfaction. Psychoeducational interventions, behavior management training, stress management, support programs, and relaxation training showed the highest impact. *Social significance:* Significant effects were reported in delaying institutionalization achieved only with multidimensional interventions. *Social validity:* All studies reported high social validity (the extent to which the intervention was found to be helpful to caregivers).	The great variability in type, dose, and intensity of interventions in studies included in this review made it difficult to attribute observed outcomes to any 1 component of active treatment conditions. Because virtually all interventions studied were multidimensional, with caregivers receiving combinations of treatment, attributing outcomes to specific causes was difficult.	Occupational therapy professionals should be aware that there is limited consensus regarding what constitutes clinical significance in caregiving intervention research. There is strong consensus that helping a caregiver with a clinical diagnosis of major depression progress to a state where he or she no longer meets criteria for this condition is a clinically significant outcome. However, the interventions included in the studies only had modest influence on depression symptoms of caregivers. Postponement of institutionalization appears to be possible with very intense, multidimensional interventions that include heavy doses of counseling, support, and education. Occupational therapy can be an integral part of such intervention, particularly in regards to environmental interventions as well as behavior management and stress management training.

Schulz, R., O'Brien, A., Czaja, S., Ory, M., Norris, R., Martire, L. M., et al. (2002). Dementia caregiver intervention research: In search of clinical significance. *Gerontologist, 42,* 589–602.

Author/Year	Study Objectives	Level/Design/Participants	Intervention and Outcome Measures	Results	Study Limitations
Smits, de Lange, Droes, Franka, Vernooij-Dassen, & Pot, 2007	This article was a review of the evidence for effects of combined intervention programs for both the informal caregiver and the person with dementia.	Level I Systematic review 25 reports related to various aspects of caregivers' mental health and burden	Intervention The included studies were classified into 3 outcome categories with respect to caregivers: mental health, burden, and competence. Outcome Measures ■ GDS ■ Zarit Burden Inventory Care Strain Questionnaire Feeling of Competence Scale ■ CES-D ■ Revised Memory and Behavioral Problems Checklist ■ Task Management Strategy Index ■ Dementia Knowledge Tests ■ Feeling of Competence Scale	Combined programs may improve some, but not all, aspects of functioning for caregivers and the person with dementia. Caregiver mental health is most likely positively affected by combined programs. Findings for other outcomes, such as depressive symptoms, well-being, and for burden, are not conclusive. Combined programs are often effective in delaying admittance to long-stay care of the care recipient.	Limited number and varying quality of available studies are of concern. Use of multiple measurement instruments for the same or similar outcome complicates interpretation of the results.	Occupational therapy personnel are qualified to direct participation or combined programs for caregivers and people with dementia. It is important that the outcome goals for these programs be clearly defined before advising client or caregiver participation in such programs. Results suggest that attention needs to be paid to the different needs of subgroups.

Smits, C., de Lange, J., Droes, R., Franka, M., Vernooij-Dassen, M., & Pot, A. (2007). Effects of combined intervention programmes for people with dementia living at home and their caregivers: A systematic review. *International Journal of Geriatric Psychiatry, 22,* 1181–1193.

Author/Year	Study Objectives	Level/Design/Participants	Intervention and Outcome Measures	Results	Study Limitations	
Thompson, Spilsbury, Hall, Birks, Barnes, & Adamson, 2007	The objective was to examine the evidence from RCTs in which technology, or individualized or group-based interventions built around the provision of support or information were evaluated.	Level I Systematic review 44 studies	Intervention Studies included in this review were categorized according to 3 types of intervention: Technology-based interventions, group-based interventions, and individual interventions. Outcome Measures Not reported	Statistically significant evidence that group-based supportive interventions affect positively on caregiver psychological morbidity. No evidence was found for the effectiveness of any other form of intervention on a range of physical and psychological health outcomes.	Outcome measures used in the studies included in the review were not reported.	Occupational therapy professionals must be aware that there is little evidence that interventions aimed at supporting or providing information to caregivers of people with dementia are uniformly effective. Such programs must be well tailored to the needs of the caregivers and be made relevant to their particular situation. However, it is recommended that caregivers be involved in supportive interventions, such as support groups, as a way to help them cope with their role. Group

(continued)

EVIDENCE TABLE: What is the effectiveness of educational and supportive strategies for caregivers of persons with dementia on the ability to maintain participation in that role? (*Contexts*) (*continued*)

Author/Year	Study Objectives	Level/Design/ Participants	Intervention and Outcome Measures	Results	Study Limitations	Implications for Occupational Therapy
Thompson, Spilsbury, Hall, Birks, Barnes, & Adamson, 2007 (cont.)						interventions underpinned by psychoeducational theoretical foundations also appear to affect depressions in caregivers.

Thompson, C., Spilsbury, K., Hall, J., Birks, Y., Barnes, C., & Adamson, J. (2007). Systematic review of information and interventions for caregivers of people with dementia. *BMC Geriatrics, 7,* 18.

Author/Year	Study Objectives	Level/Design/ Participants	Intervention and Outcome Measures	Results	Study Limitations	Implications for Occupational Therapy
Winter & Gitlin, 2006	The objective was to evaluate the feasibility and effectiveness of professionally led, telephone-based support groups for female family caregivers of community-dwelling dementia patients.	Level I RCT\n\nParticipants\n103 women caregivers, all age ≥ 50 (mean age 66.6), who had provided a minimum of 6 mo of care to a relative with AD and who had access to a telephone for > 1 hr each week\n\nThe majority (68.3%) of caregivers were White, and the remaining were African-American.	Intervention\nAfter an initial interview, participants were randomly assigned to intervention or control. Intervention consisted of participation in a telephone-based support group over 6 mo (possible 26 sessions). Telesupport groups were conducted by trained social workers who used conference-calling technology to link 5 caregivers per group for 1 hr weekly. Initially, facilitators focused on building group cohesion and caregivers expressed emotions and shared coping strategies, including cognitive reframing and practical approaches to organizing care routines. They also assisted each other in problem solving and shared educational resources.	No large or statistically significant differences between experimental and control group participants were reported at 6 mo on the outcome measures.\n\nAll caregivers scored high in depression, but older caregivers in the telesupport groups scored slightly lower, suggesting more benefit to this group.\n\nRace was not found to be associated with any 6 mo outcomes.\n\nSession attendance was not found to be associated with depression, caregiver burden, or gains at 6 mo.	Limitations were small sample size and nonrepresentative sample, which excluded other ethnic groups and male caregivers.	Telesupport groups seemed to provide limited benefit mostly to older (age 65+) caregivers. Occupational therapy professionals may consider inclusion of such intervention as part of an overall program if it appears that the caregiver is relatively isolated and has greater need for social contact.

The control group received
no treatment.

Outcome Measures
- Centers for
  Epidemiological Studies
  Depression Scale
- Zarit Burden Scale
- Gains Through Group
  Involvement Scale

Winter, L., & Gitlin, L. N. (2006). Evaluation of a telephone-based support group intervention for female caregivers of community-dwelling individuals with dementia. *American Journal of Alzheimer's Disease and Other Dementias, 21,* 391–397.

Note. AAL-AD = Affect and Activity Limitation-Alzheimer's Disease Assessment; ABMI = Agitation Behavior Mapping Instrument; AD = Alzheimer's disease; ADAS = Alzheimer's Disease Assessment Scale; ADAS-Cog = Alzheimer's Disease Assessment Scale–cognitive subscale; ADLs = activities of daily living; AFG = attention-focusing group; AIF = Assessment of Instrumental Function; AIS = Abbreviated Injury Scale; AMPS = Assessment of Motor and Process Skills; ANCOVA = analysis of covariance; ANOVA = analysis of variance; BACE = Balancing Arousal Controls Excesses; BCRS = Brief Cognitive Rating scale; BEHAVE = Behavioral Pathology in Alzheimer's Disease Rating Scale; BMD = Behavior and Mood Disturbance scale; BMI = body mass index; BRS = Behavior Rating Scale; CANDEX = Cambridge Examination for Mental Disorders of the Elderly; CAPE = Clifton Assessment Procedures for the Elderly; CAS = Cognitive Assessment Scale; CDR = Clinical Dementia Rating; CES-D = Center for Epidemiological Studies Depression scale; CMAI = Cohen-Mansfield Agitation Inventory; CNA = certified nursing assistant; COPM = Canadian Occupational Performance Measure; CST = cognitive stimulation therapy; DAT = Dementia of the Alzheimer Type; DSCU = Dementia Special Care Unit; DSM = *Diagnostic and Statistical Manual;* FAC = Functional Abilities Checklist; FIMs = Functional Independence Measures; GDS = Geriatric Depression scale; GHQ = General Health Questionnaire; IADLs = instrumental activities of daily living; IDDD = Interview of deterioration in daily activities in dementia; ITT = intention to treat; *M* = mean; MDS = minimum data set; MMSE = Mini-Mental Status Examination; NINCDS-ADRDA = National Institute of Neurological and Communicative Disorders and Stroke and the Alzheimer's Disease and Related Disorders Association; NITE-AD = Nighttime Insomnia Treatment and Education for Alzheimer's Disease; NS = no significant; NPI = Neuropsychiatric Inventory; SI = sensory integration; RHR = resting heart rate; OARS = Older Americans Resources and Services Multidimensional Assessment Questionnaire; OBS Scale = Organic Brain Syndrome scale; PSMS = Physical Self-Maintenance scale; QoL-AD = Quality of Life-Alzheimer's Disease; RCT = randomized controlled trial; REACH = Resources for Enhancing Alzheimer's Caregiver Health; REHAB = Rehabilitation Evaluation Hall and Baker; RMBPC = Revised Memory and Behavior Problems Checklist; SCU = special care unit; *SD* = standard deviation; TAP = Tailored Activity Program; WIB = Well-Being/Ill-Being scale.

Appendix F.
Driving and Community Mobility for Persons With Alzheimer's Disease

Drivers with Alzheimer's disease are at risk for motor vehicle crashes and poor performance of road tests at a rate higher than older drivers without Alzheimer's disease (Drachman & Swearer, 1993; Duchek et al., 2003; Fitten et al., 1995). This risk has particular significance because driving and community mobility issues occupy a central place in the lives of older adults and their families and friends. *Community mobility*, which includes driving, is defined as "moving around in the community, and using public or private transportation, such as driving, walking, bicycling, or accessing or riding in buses, taxi cabs or other transportation systems" (AOTA, 2008b, p. 631). Although driving and community mobility are important in their own right, they are also significant because of their influence on facilitating or hindering performance in other areas of occupation, including leisure, social participation, and other instrumental activities of daily living (Stav, Hunt, & Arbesman, 2006). In addition, reports of driving cessation as an independent risk factor for depressive symptoms in elderly people (Marottoli et al., 1997; Ragland, Satariano, & MacLeod, 2005) point to the importance of driving in the lives of older adults.

The following questions arise related to the impact of Alzheimer's disease and driving:

- Which cognitive and visual skills affected in Alzheimer's disease are of importance for driving performance?
- Does the stage of Alzheimer's disease determine whether or not someone is able to drive?
- Are compensatory strategies for driving an effective approach for people with Alzheimer's disease?

- What is the appropriate period for a follow-up evaluation for a person with Alzheimer's disease as he or she progresses through stages of the disease?

Research indicates that, separate from general age-related changes, visual perception, processing, attention, verbal and visual memory, and executive function are the components of cognitive and visual skills needed for driving performance that are affected by Alzheimer's disease (Uc et al., 2005). According to the results of focus groups consisting of health professionals, transportation and law enforcement professionals, current and former drivers with Alzheimer's disease, and family caregivers of the drivers, participants felt, with only a few exceptions, that mild Alzheimer's disease alone did not preclude driving (Perkinson et al., 2005). Findings from longitudinal quantitative studies (Duchek et al., 2003; Ott et al., 2008) reflect this feeling and indicate that although cognitive changes in early Alzheimer's disease may result in higher risk of motor vehicle crashes and poor driving performance, some individuals with early Alzheimer's disease may continue to drive safely. Although no studies were found in a systematic review to evaluate the effect of compensatory strategies on driving performance of older adults with Alzheimer's disease (Man-Son-Hing et al., 2007), other studies point to best practice for occupational therapy practitioners working with adults with mild Alzheimer's disease. Evidence is limited on the optimal length of time for a follow-up evaluation of driving performance for those with Alzheimer's disease. Two systematic reviews of the evidence, however, recommend a 6-month follow-up (Adler, Rottunda, &

Dysken, 2005; Molnar, Patel, Marshall, Man-Son-Hing, & Wilson, 2006). Adler and colleagues (2005) recommended neuropsychological tests that examine visual–spatial skills, attention, and reaction time to examine driving performance in this population. According to Man-Son-Hing and colleagues (2007), evaluation of these skills by health professionals in combination with an on-road driving evaluation is the most appropriate method to determine fitness to drive for persons with mild Alzheimer's disease. The *Occupational Therapy Practice Guidelines for Driving and Community Mobility for Older Adults* (Stav et al., 2006) provides additional information on driving assessment and intervention for older adults.

■ ■ ■

References

Abraham, I. L. (2005). Dementia and Alzheimer's disease: A practical orientation. *Nursing Clinics of North America, 41,* 119–127.

Abramowicz, M. (Ed.). (2007). Drugs for cognitive loss and dementia. *Treatment Guidelines From the Medical Letter, 5*(54), 9–14.

Accreditation Council for Occupational Therapy Education. (2007a). Accreditation standards for a doctoral-degree-level educational program for the occupational therapist. *American Journal of Occupational Therapy, 61,* 641–651.

Accreditation Council for Occupational Therapy Education. (2007b). Accreditation standards for a master's-degree-level educational program for the occupational therapist. *American Journal of Occupational Therapy, 61,* 652–661.

Accreditation Council for Occupational Therapy Education. (2007c). Accreditation standards for an educational program for the occupational therapy assistant. *American Journal of Occupational Therapy, 61,* 662–671.

Acton, G. J., & Kang, J. (2001). Interventions to reduce the burden of caregiving for an adult with dementia: A meta-analysis. *Research in Nursing and Health, 24*(5), 349–360.

Adler, G., Rottunda, S., & Dysken, M. (2005). The older driver with dementia: An updated literature review. *Journal of Safety Research, 36,* 399–407.

Administration on Aging. (2009). *AoA programs.* Retrieved November 6, 2009, from www.aoa.gov /AoARoot/AoA_Programs/index.aspx

Agency for Healthcare Research and Quality, U.S. Preventive Services Task Force. (2009). *Standard recommendation language.* Retrieved February 14, 2009, from http://www.ahrq.gov/clinic/uspstf/standard.htm

Alessi, C. A., Martin, J. L., Webber, A. P., Kim, E. C., Harker, J. O., & Josephson, K. R. (2005). Randomized, controlled trial of a non-pharmacological intervention to improve abnormal sleep/wake patterns in nursing home residents. *Journal of the American Geriatrics Society, 53,* 803–810.

Allen, C. K., Austin, S. L. David, S. K., Earhart, C. A., McCraith, D. B., & Riska-Williams, L. (2007). *Manual for the Allen Cognitive Level Screen–5 (ACLS–5) and Large Allen Cognitive Level Screen (LACLS–5).* Camarillo, CA: ACLS and LACLS Committee.

Allen, C., Earhart, C. A., & Blue, T. (1992). *Occupational therapy treatment goals for the physically and cognitively disabled.* Rockville, MD: American Occupational Therapy Association.

Allen, C., & Reyner, A. (2008). *How to start using the Allen Diagnostic Module* (9th ed.). Cochester, CT: S&S Worldwide.

Altus, D. E., Engelman, K. K., & Mathews, R. M. (2002). Using family-style meals to increase participation and communication in persons with dementia. *Journal of Gerontological Nursing, 28,* 47–53.

Alzheimer's Association. (2008). *Safety center.* Retrieved November 6, 2009, from www.alz.org/safetycenter/we_ can_help_safety_medicalert_safereturn.asp

Alzheimer's Association. (2009a). *2009 Alzheimer's disease facts and figures.* Retrieved November 25, 2009, from www.alz.org/alzheimers_disease_facts_figures.asp

Alzheimer's Association. (2009b). *Comfort zone.* Retrieved November 6, 2009, from www.alz.org/comfortzone/

Alzheimer's Association. (2009c). *Stages of Alzheimer's.* Retrieved January 18, 2010, from http://www.alz.org/alzheimers_disease_stages_of_alzheimers.asp

Alzheimer's Association & National Alliance for Caregiving. (2004). *Families care: Alzheimer's caregiving in the United States.* Retrieved November 25, 2009, from www.alz.org/national/documents/report_familiescare.pdf

American Academy of Family Physicians. (2008). *Sleep changes in older adults.* Retrieved November 25, 2009, from http://familydoctor.org/online/famdocen/home/seniors/common-older/386.html

American Academy of Neurology. (2008). *AAN Guideline summary for clinicians: Detection, diagnosis, and management of dementia.* Retrieved November 25, 2009, from www.aan.com/professionals/practice/pdfs/dementia_guideline.pdf

American Occupational Therapy Association. (1979). Uniform terminology for occupational therapy. *Occupational Therapy News, 35*(11), 1–8.

American Occupational Therapy Association. (1989). Uniform terminology for occupational therapy (2nd ed.). *American Journal of Occupational Therapy, 43,* 808–815.

American Occupational Therapy Association. (1994). Uniform terminology for occupational therapy (3rd ed.). *American Journal of Occupational Therapy, 48,* 1047–1054.

American Occupational Therapy Association. (2002). Occupational therapy practice framework: Domain and process. *American Journal of Occupational Therapy, 56,* 609–639.

American Occupational Therapy Association. (2006). Policy 1.44: Categories of occupational therapy personnel. In *Policy manual* (2007 ed., pp. 33–34). Bethesda, MD: Author.

American Occupational Therapy Association. (2008a). Guidelines for documentation of occupational therapy. *American Journal of Occupational Therapy, 62,* 684–690.

American Occupational Therapy Association. (2008b). Occupational therapy practice framework: Domain and process (2nd ed.). *American Journal of Occupational Therapy, 62,* 625–683.

American Occupational Therapy Association. (2009). Guidelines for supervision, roles, and responsibilities during the delivery of occupational therapy services. *American Journal of Occupational Therapy, 63,* 797–803.

American Psychiatric Association. (2000). *Diagnostic and statistical manual of mental disorders* (4th ed., text rev.). Washington, DC: Author.

Avila, R., Bottino, C. M., Carvalho, I. A., Santos, C. B., Seral, C., & Miotto, E. C. (2004). Neuropsychological rehabilitation of memory deficits and activities of daily living in patients with Alzheimer's disease: A pilot study. *Brazilian Journal of Medical and Biological Research, 37,* 1721–1729.

Aykan, H. (2003). Effect of childlessness on nursing home and home health care use. *Journal of Aging and Social Policy, 15*(1), 33–53.

Baillon, S., van Diepen, E., Prettyman, R., Redman, J., Rooke, N., & Campbell, R. (2004). Comparison of the effects of Snoezelen and reminiscence therapy on the agitated behaviour of patients with dementia. *International Journal of Geriatric Psychiatry, 19*(11), 1047–1052.

Baillon, S., van Diepen, E., Prettyman, R., Rooke, N., Redman, J., & Campbell, R. (2005). Variability in response to older people with dementia to both Snoezelen and reminiscence. *British Journal of Occupational Therapy, 68*(8), 367–374.

Baker, R., Bell, S., Baker, E., Gibson, S., Holloway, J., Pearce, R., et al. (2001). A randomized controlled trial of the effects of multi-sensory stimulation (MSS) for people with dementia. *British Journal of Clinical Psychology, 40*(1), 81–96.

Baker, R., Dowling, Z., Wareing, L. A., Dawson, J., & Assey, J. (1997). Snoezelen: Its long-term and short-term effects on older people with dementia. *British Journal of Occupational Therapy, 60*(5), 213–218.

Bank, A. L., Argüelles, S., Rubert, M., Eisdorfer, C., & Czaja, S. J. (2006). The value of telephone support groups among ethnically diverse caregivers of persons with dementia. *Gerontologist, 46,* 134–138.

Baron, K., Kielhofner, G., Iyenger, A., Goldhammer, V., & Wokenski, J. (2006). *The Occupational Self-Assessment* (OSA; Version 2.2). Chicago: Model of Human Occupation Clearinghouse, Department of Occupational Therapy, College of Applied Health Sciences, University of Illinois.

Bass-Haugen, J., Henderson, M. L., Larson, B. A., & Matuska, K. (2005). Occupational issues of concern in populations. In C. H. Christiansen & C. M. Baum (Eds.), *Occupational therapy: Performance, participation, and well-being* (pp. 167–187). Thorofare, NJ: Slack.

Baum, C. M., Connor, L. T., Morrison, T., Hahn, M., Dromerick, A. W., & Edwards. D. F. (2008). Reliability, validity, and clinical utility of the executive function performance test: A measure of executive function in a sample of people with stroke. *American Journal of Occupational Therapy, 62*(4), 446–455.

Baum, C., & Edwards D. F. (1993). Cognitive performance in senile dementia of the Alzheimer's type: The Kitchen Task Assessment. *American Journal of Occupational Therapy, 47*(5), 431–436.

Baum, C. M., Morrison, T., Hahn, M., & Edwards, D. F. (2003). *Executive Function Performance Test.* St. Louis, MO: Washington University.

Beattie, E. R., Algase, D. L., & Song, J. (2004). Keeping wandering nursing home residents at the table: Improv-

ing food intake using a behavioral communication intervention. *Aging and Mental Health, 8,* 109–116.

Bendall, M. J., Bassey, E. J., & Pearson, M. B. (1989). Factors affecting walking speed of elderly people. *Age and Aging, 18,* 327–332.

Bennett, D. A., Wilson, R. S., Schneider, J. A., Evans, D. A., Mendes de Leon, C. F., Arnold, S. E., et al. (2003). Education modifies the relation of AD pathology to level of cognitive function in older persons. *Neurology, 60,* 1909–1915.

Bentham, P., & LaFontaine, J. (2005). Services for younger people with dementia. *Psychiatry, 4*(2), 100–103.

Berg, K. O., Wood-Dauphinee, J. I., & Williams, B. (1992). Measuring balance in the elderly: Validation of an instrument. *Canadian Journal of Public Health, 83*(Supp. 12), S7–S11.

Bimesser, L. R. (1997). Treating dementia. *OT Practice, 2*(6), 16–21.

Blieszner, R., Roberto, K. A., Wilcox, K. L., Barham, E. J., & Winston, B. L. (2007). Dimensions of ambiguous loss in couples coping with mild cognitive impairment. *Family Relations, 56*(2), 196–209.

Bliwise, D. L. (2004). Sleep disorders in Alzheimer's disease and other dementias. *Clinical Cornerstone, 6*(1A), S16–S28.

Bourgeois, M. S., & Mason, L. A. (1996). Memory wallet intervention in an adult day-care setting. *Behavioral Interventions, 11,* 3–18.

Boylston, E., Ryan, C., Brown, C., & Westfall, B. (1995). Increasing oral intake in dementia patients by altering food texture. *American Journal of Alzheimer's Disease, 10,* 37–39.

Brodaty, H., Green, A., & Koschera, A. (2003). Meta-analysis of psychosocial interventions for caregivers of people with dementia. *Journal of the American Geriatrics Society, 51*(5), 657–664.

Brooker, D., & Duce, L. (2000). Well-being and activity in dementia: A comparison of group reminiscence therapy, structured goal-directed group activity and unstructured time. *Aging and Mental Health, 4,* 354–358.

Brookmeyer, R. (2006). Dementia. *Geriatric Cognitive Disorders, 21,* 175–181.

Brookmeyer, R., Ziegler-Graham, K., Johnson, E., & Arrighi, H. M. (2007). *Forecasting the global burden of Alzheimer's disease.* Retrieved January 18, 2010, from http://www.bepress.com/jhubiostat/paper130.

Brown, C. (2009). Ecological models in occupational therapy. In E. B. Crepeau, E. S. Cohn, & B. A. Boyt Schell (Eds.), *Willard and Spackman's occupational therapy* (11th ed., pp. 435–461). Baltimore: Lippincott Williams & Wilkins.

Brown, C., & Dunn, W. (2002). *Adolescent/Adult Sensory Profile.* San Antonio, TX: Psychological Corporation.

Brown, S. M., Humphry, R., & Taylor, E. (1996). A model of the nature of family–therapist relationships: Implications for education. *American Journal of Occupational Therapy, 51,* 597–603.

Buchman, A. S. (2006). Body mass index in older persons is associated with Alzheimer disease pathology. *Neurology, 67*(11), 1949–1954.

Buettner, L. L. (1999). Simple pleasures: A multilevel sensorimotor intervention for nursing home residents with dementia. *American Journal of Alzheimer's Disease, 14,* 41–52.

Burns, T. (1991, 1996). *Cognitive performance test (CPT): A measure of cognitive capacity for the performance of routine tasks.* Minneapolis, MN: Geriatric Research, Education and Clinical Center, Minneapolis VA Medical Center.

Burns, T. (2006) *Cognitive Performance Test (CPT): 2006 manual.* Pequannock, NJ: Maddak.

Burns, T., Mortimer, J., & Merchak, P. (1994). Cognitive Performance Test: A new approach to functional assessment in Alzheimer's disease. *Journal of Geriatric Psychiatry and Neurology, 7,* 46–54.

Burns, R., Nichols, L. O., Martindale-Adams, J., Graney, M. J., & Lummus, A. (2003). Primary care interventions for dementia caregivers: 2-year outcomes from the REACH study. *Gerontologist, 43*(4), 547–555.

Caselli, R. J., Beach, T. G., Yaari, R., & Reiman, E. M. (2006). Alzheimer's disease a century later. *Journal of Clinical Psychiatry, 67,* 1784–1800.

Centers for Medicare and Medicaid Services. (2008). *Medicare benefit policy manual.* Retrieved June 28, 2009, from www.cms.hhs.gov/manuals/Downloads/bp102c15.pdf

Christiansen, C. H., Baum, C. M., & Bass-Haugen, J. (Eds.). (2005). *Occupational therapy: Performance, participation, and well-being* (3rd ed.). Thorofare, NJ: Slack.

Chung, J. C. C. (2004). Activity participation and well-being of people with dementia in long-term-care settings. *OTJR: Occupation, Participation and Health, 24,* 22–31.

Chung, J. C. C., & Lai, C. K. (2002). Snoezelen for dementia. *Cochrane Database of Systematic Reviews: Reviews 2002, Issue 4.*

Chung, J. C. C., & Lai, C. K. Y. (2006). Snoezelen for dementia. *Cochrane Library,* (4), (CD003152).

Clair, A. A., & Ebberts, A. (1997). The effects of music therapy on interactions between family caregivers and their care receivers with late-stage dementia. *Journal of Music Therapy, 34*(3), 148–164.

Clarfield, A. M. (2003). The decreasing prevalence of reversible dementias. *Archives of Internal Medicine, 163,* 2219–2229.

Cohen-Mansfield, J., & Werner, P. (1998). The effects of an enhanced environment on nursing home residents who pace. *Gerontologist, 38*(2), 199–208.

Colling, K. B., & Buettner, L. L. (2002). Simple pleasures: Interventions from the need-driven dementia-compromised behavior model. *Journal of Gerontological Nursing, 28,* 16–20.

Congressional Budget Office. (2004). *Financing long-term care for the elderly.* Washington, DC: Author. Retrieved June 15, 2004, from www.cbo.gov/showdoc.cfm?index=5400&sequence=0

Cooke, D. D., McNally, L., Mulligan, K. T., Harrison, M. J., & Newman, S. P. (2001). Psychosocial interventions for caregivers of people with dementia: A systematic review. *Aging and Mental Health, 5*(2), 120–135.

Corcoran, M. (1999). *Occupational therapy practice guidelines for adults with Alzheimer's disease.* Bethesda, MD: American Occupational Therapy Association.

Corcoran, M. A., Gitlin, L. N., Levy, L., Eckhardt, S., Vause Earland, T., Shaw, G., et al. (2002). An occupational therapy home-based intervention to address dementia-related problems identified by family caregivers. *Alzheimer's Care Quarterly, 3,* 82–89.

Coyne, M. L., & Hoskins, L. (1997). Improving eating behaviors in dementia using behavioral strategies. *Clinical Nursing Research, 6*(3), 275–290.

Crispi, E. L., & Heitner, G. (2002). An activity-based intervention for caregivers and residents with dementia in nursing homes. *Activities, Adaptation, and Aging, 26,* 61–72.

Curry, L. C., Walker, C., & Hogstel, M. O. (2006) Educational needs of employed family caregivers of older adults: Evaluation of a workplace project. *Geriatric Nursing, 27*(3), 166–173.

de Leon, M. J., & Klunk, W. (2006). Biomarkers for the early diagnosis of Alzheimer's disease. *Lancet Neurology, 5*(3), 198–199.

Detweiler, M. B., Kim, K. Y., & Taylor, B. Y. (2005). Focused supervision of high-risk fall dementia patients: A simple method to reduce fall incidence and severity. *American Journal of Alzheimer's Disease and Other Dementias, 20,* 97–104.

Dickinson, J. I., McLain-Kark, J., & Marshall-Baker, A. (1995). The effects of visual barriers on exiting behavior in a dementia care unit. *Gerontologist, 35*(1), 127–130.

Dilworth-Anderson, P., Williams, I. C., & Gibson, B. E. (2002). Issues of race, ethnicity, and culture in caregiving research: A 20 year review (1980–2000). *Gerontologist, 42,* 237–272.

Donovan, C., & Dupuis, M. (2000). Specialized care unit: Family and staff perceptions of significant elements. *Geriatric Nursing, 21,* 30–33.

Doody, R. S., Stevens, J. C., Beck, C., Dubinsky, R. M., Kaye, J. A., Gwyther, L., et al. (2001). Practice parameter: Management of dementia (an evidence-based review). Report of the Quality Standards Subcommittee of the American Academy of Neurology. *Neurology, 56,* 1154–1166.

Doody, R. S., Strehlow, L., Massman, P. J., Feher, E. P., Clark, C., & Roy, J. R. (1999). Baylor Profound Mental Status Examination: A brief staging measure for profoundly demented Alzheimer disease patients. *Alzheimer Disease and Associated Disorders, 13*(1), 53–59.

Dooley, N. R., & Hinojosa, J. (2004). Improving quality of life for persons with Alzheimer's disease and their family caregivers: Brief occupational therapy intervention. *American Journal of Occupational Therapy, 58,* 561–569.

Drachman, D. A., & Swearer, J. M. (1993). Driving and Alzheimer's disease: The risk of crashes. *Neurology, 43,* 2448–2456.

Drane, D. L., Yuspeh, R. L., Huthwaite, J. S., Klingler, L. K., Foster, L. M., Mrazik, M., et al. (2003). Healthy older adult performance on a modified version of the Cognistat (NCSE): Demographic issues and preliminary normative data. *Journal of Clinical and Experimental Neuropsychology, 25*(1), 133–144.

Dubinsky, R. M., Stein, A. C., & Lyons, K. (2000). Practice parameter: Risk of driving and Alzheimer's diseases (an evidence-based review): Report of the Quality Standards Subcommitteee of the American Academy of Neurology. *Neurology, 54,* 2205–2211.

Duchek, J. M., Carr, D. B., Hunt, L. A., Roe, C. M., Xiong, C., Shah, K., et al. (2003). Longitudinal driving performance in early-stage dementia of the Alzheimer type. *Journal of the American Geriatrics Society, 51,* 1342–1347.

Dunn, W., Brown, C., & Youngstrom, M. J. (2003). Ecological model of occupation. In P. Kramer, J. Hinojosa, & C. B. Royeen (Eds.), *Perspectives in human occupation* (pp. 222–263). Philadelphia: Lippincott Williams & Wilkins.

Dyer, C. B., Pavlick, V. N., Pace-Murphy, K., & Hyman, D. J. (2000). The high prevalence of depression and dementia in elder abuse and neglect. *Journal of the American Geriatric Society, 48*(2), 205–208.

Elmståhl, S., Annerstedt, L., & Åhlund, O. (1997). How should a group living unit for demented elderly be designed to decrease psychiatric symptoms? *Alzheimer Disease and Associated Disorders, 11*(1), 47–52.

Engelhart, C., Eisenstein, N., Johnson, V., Wolf, J., Williamson, J., Steitz, D., et al. (1999). Factor structure of the Neurobehavioral Cognitive Status Exam (Cognistat) in healthy, and psychiatrically and neurologically impaired, elderly adults. *Clinical Neuropsychology, 13*(1), 109–111.

Eustice, S., Roe, B., & Paterson, J. (2000). Prompted voiding for the management of urinary incontinence in adults. *Cochrane Database of Systematic Reviews, 2,* CD002113. doi: 10.1002/14651858.CD002113

Fagan, L. (2002). Strategies to promote independence in self-feeding for persons with dementia. *Gerontology Special Interest Section Quarterly, 25*(2), 1–3.

Fillit, H., & Hill, J. (2005). Economics of dementia and pharmacoeconomics of dementia therapy. *American Journal of Geriatric Pharmacotherapy, 3*(1), 39–49.

Fischer, A. G. (1997). *Assessment of Motor and Process Skills* (2nd ed.). Fort Collins, CO: Three Star.

Fitten, L. J., Perryman, K. M., Wilkinson, C. J., Little, R. J., Burns, M. M., Pachana, N., et al. (1995). Alzheimer and vascular dementias and driving: A prospective road and laboratory study. *JAMA, 273,* 1360–1365.

Fitzsimmons, S., & Buettner, L. L. (2003). A therapeutic cooking program for older adults with dementia: Effects on agitation and apathy. *American Journal of Recreation Therapy, 2,* 23–33.

Folstein, M. F., Folstein, S. E., & McHugh, P. R. (1975). Mini-Mental State: A practical method for grading the cognitive state of patients for the clinician. *Journal of Psychiatric Research, 12,* 196–198.

Garwick, A. W., Detzner, D., & Boss, P. (1994). Family perceptions of living with Alzheimer's disease. *Family Process, 33,* 327–340.

Gelinas, I., Gauthier, L., McIntyre, M., & Gauthier, S. (1999). Development of a functional measure for persons with Alzheimer's disease: The Disability Assessment for Dementia. *American Journal of Occupational Therapy, 53*(5), 471–481.

Gibson, M. C., MacLean, J., Borrie, M., & Geiger, J. (2004). Orientation behaviors in residents relocated to a redesigned dementia care unit. *American Journal of Alzheimer's Disease and Other Dementias, 19*(1), 45–49.

Gitlin, L. N., Corcoran, M., Winter, L., Boyce, A., & Hauck, W. W. (2001). A randomized, controlled trial of a home environment intervention: Effect on efficacy and upset in caregivers and on daily functioning of persons with dementia. *Gerontologist, 41,* 4–14.

Gitlin, L. N., Hauck, W. W., Dennis, M. P., & Winter, L. (2005). Maintenance of effects of the Home Environmental Skill-building Program for family caregivers and individuals with Alzheimer's disease and related disorders. *Journal of Gerontology Series A: Biological and Medical Sciences, 60*(3), 368–374.

Gitlin, L. N., Schinfeld, S., Winter, L., Corcoran, M., Boyce A. A., & Hauck, W. (2002). Evaluating home environments of persons with dementia: Interrater reliability and validity of the Home Environmental Assessment Protocol (HEAP). *Disability and Rehabilitation, 24*(1–3), 59–71.

Gitlin, L., Winter, L., Burke, J., Chernett, N., Dennis, M., & Hauck, W. (2008). Tailored activities to manage neuropsychiatric behaviors in persons with dementia and reduce caregiver burden: A randomized pilot study. *American Journal of Geriatric Psychiatry, 16*(3), 229–239.

Goetz, G. (Ed.). (2003). *Textbook of clinical neurology* (2nd ed.). St. Louis, MO: W. B. Saunders.

Goldman, L. (Ed.). (2004). *Cecil textbook of medicine* (22nd ed.). St. Louis, MO: W. B. Saunders.

Gotell, E., Brown, S., & Ekman, S. L. (2002). Caregiver singing and background music in dementia care. *Western Journal of Nursing Research, 24,* 195–216.

Gotell, E., Brown, S., & Ekman, S. (2003). Influence of caregiver singing and background music on posture, movement, and sensory awareness in dementia care. *International Psychogeriatrics, 15*(4), 411–430.

Graff, M., Adang, E., Vernooij-Dassen, M., Dekker, J., Jomsson, L., Thijssen, M., et al. (2008). Community occupational therapy for older patients with dementia and their caregivers: Cost effectiveness study. *British Medical Journal, 336,* 134–138.

Graff, M. J. L., Vernooij-Dassen, M. J. M., Hoefnagels, W. H., Dekker, J., & de Witte, L. P. (2003). Occupational therapy at home for older individuals with mild to moderate cognitive impairments and their primary caregivers: A pilot study. *Occupational Therapy Journal of Research, 23,* 155–163.

Graff, M. J. L., Vernooij-Dassen, M. J. M., Thijssen, M., Dekker, J., Hoefnagels, W. H. L., & Rikkert, M. G. M. (2006). Community-based occupational therapy for patients with dementia and their caregivers: Randomized controlled trial. *British Medical Journal, 333,* 1196–1201.

Graff, M., Vernooij-Dassen, M., Thijssen, M., Dekker, J., Hoefnagels, W., & Rikkert, M. G. (2007). Effects of community occupational therapy on quality of life, mood, and health status in dementia patients and their caregivers: A randomized controlled trial. *Journal of Gerontology: Medical Sciences, 62A*(9), 1002–1009.

GRECC Caregiver Materials. (1996). Minneapolis, MN: Dementia Care Clinic, GRECC Center, Minneapolis VA Medical Center.

Gwyther, L. P. (1995). When the family system is not one voice: Conflict in caregiving families. *Journal of Case Management, 4*(4), 150–155.

Hauer, K., Becker, C., Lindemann, U., & Beyer, N. (2006). Effectiveness of physical training on motor performance and fall prevention in cognitively impaired older persons: A systematic review. *American Journal of Physical Medicine and Rehabilitation, 85,* 847–857.

Heimann, N. E., Allen, C. K., & Yerxa, E. J. (1989). The Routine Task Inventory: A tool for describing the functional behavior of the cognitively disabled. *Occupational Therapy Practice, 1,* 67–74.

Hepburn, K., Lewis, M., Narayan, S., Center, B., Tornatore, J., Bremer, K., et al. (2005). Partners in caregiving: A psychoeducation program affecting dementia family caregivers' distress and caregiving outlook. *Clinical Gerontologist, 29*(1), 53–69.

Hepburn, K. W., Tornatore, J., Center, B., & Ostwald, S. W. (2001). Dementia family caregiver training: Affecting beliefs about caregiving and caregiver outcomes. *Journal of the American Geriatrics Society, 49*(4), 450–457.

Heyn, P. (2003). The effect of a multisensory exercise program on engagement, behavior, and selected physiological indexes in persons with dementia. *American Journal of Alzheimer's Disease and Other Dementias, 18*(4), 247–251.

Holm, M. B., & Rogers, J. C. (1999). Functional assessment: The Performance Assessment of Self-care Skills (PASS). In B. J. Hemphill (Ed.), *Assessments in occupational therapy mental health: An integrative approach* (pp. 117–124). Thorofare, NJ: Slack.

Hope, K. (1998). The effects of multisensory environments on older people with dementia. *Journal of Psychiatric and Mental Health Nursing, 5,* 377–385.

Hosaka, T., & Sugiyama, Y. (2003) Structured intervention in family caregivers of the demented elderly and changes in their immune function. *Psychiatry and Clinical Neurosciences, 57*(2), 147–151.

Hua, X., Leow, A. D., Lee, S., Klunder, A. D., Toga, A. W., Lepore, N., et al. (2008). 3D characterization of brain atrophy in Alzheimer's disease and mild cognitive impairment using tensor-based morphometry. *Neuroimage, 41*(1), 19–34.

Huang, H. L., Lotus Shyu, Y. I., Chen, M. C., Chen, S. T., & Lin, L. C. (2003). A pilot study on a home-based caregiver training program for improving caregiver self-efficacy and decreasing the behavioral problems of elders with dementia in Taiwan. *International Journal of Geriatric Psychiatry, 18*(4), 337–345.

Hutchinson, S., Leger-Krall, S., & Wilson, H. S. (1996). Toileting: A biobehavioral challenge in Alzheimer's dementia care. *Journal of Gerontological Nursing, 22,* 18–27.

Iwama, M. (2006). *The Kawa model: Culturally relevant occupational therapy.* New York: Church Livingstone/ Elsevier.

Jecker, N. S. (2001). Family caregiving: A problem of justice. In D. N. Weisstub, D. D. Thomasma, S. Gauthier, & G. F. Tomossy (Eds.), *Aging: Caring for our elders* (pp. 19–28). Boston: Kluwer Academic.

Jensen, J., Nyberg, L., Gustafson, Y., & Lundin-Olsson, L. (2003). Fall and injury prevention in residential care: Effects in residents with higher and lower levels of cognition. *Journal of the American Geriatrics Society, 51,* 627–635.

Jensen, J., Nyberg, L., Rosendahl, E., Gustafson, Y., & Lundin-Olsson, L. (2004). Effects of a fall prevention program including exercise on mobility and falls in frail older people living in residential care facilities. *Aging Clinical and Experimental Research, 16*(4), 283–292.

Karagiozis, H., Gray, S., Sacco, J., Shapiro, M., & Kawas, C. (1998). The Direct Assessment of Functional Abilities (DAFA): A comparison to an indirect measure of instrumental activities of daily living. *Gerontologist, 38*(1), 113–121.

Kasper, J. D., Steinbach, U., & Andrews, J. (1990, February). *Factors associated with ending caregiving among informal caregivers to the functionally and cognitively impaired elderly population.* Washington, DC: U.S. Department of Health and Human Services. Retrieved March 10, 2004, from http://aspe.hhs.gov/daltcp/ reports/factores.htm

Katz, N. (2006). *Routine Task Inventory–RTI–E manual, prepared and elaborated on the basis of Allen, C.K.* (Unpublished manuscript).

Katz, N., Itzkovich, M., Averbuch, S., & Elazar, B. (1989). Loewenstein Occupational Therapy Cognitive Assessment (LOTCA) Battery for Brain-Injured Patients: Reliability and validity. *American Journal of Occupational Therapy, 43*(3), 184–192.

Keith, R. A., Granger, C. V., Hamilton, B. B., & Sherwin, F. S. (1987). The Functional Independence Measure: A new tool for rehabilitation. *Advances in Clinical Rehabilitation, 1,* 6–18.

Kelley, B. J., & Petersen, R. C. (2007). Alzheimer's disease and mild cognitive impairment. *Neurology Clinics, 25,* 577–609.

Kelley, R. E., & Minagar, A. (2004). Memory complaints and dementia. *Primary Care Clinical Office Practice, 31,* 129–148.

Kielhofner, G. (2008). *Model of Human Occupation* (4th ed). Baltimore: Wolters Kluwer.

Kincaid, C., & Peacock, J. R. (2003). Effect of a wall mural on decreasing four types of door-testing behaviors. *Journal of Applied Gerontology, 22*(1), 76–88.

Kirschstein, R. (2000). *Disease-specific estimates of direct and indirect costs of illness and NIH support: Fiscal year 2000 update.* Washington, DC: U.S. Department of Health and Human Services.

Kizony, R., & Katz, N. (2002). Relationships between cognitive abilities and the process scale and skills of the Assessment of Motor and Process Skills (AMPS) in patients with stroke. *OTJR: Occupation, Participation and Health, 22*(2), 82–92.

Kohlman Thompson, L. (1992). *The Kohlman Evaluation of Living Skills.* Rockville, MD: American Occupational Therapy Association.

Kolanowski, A. (2001). Capturing interests: Therapeutic recreation activities for persons with dementia. *Therapeutic Recreation Journal, 35,* 220–235.

Koppel, R. (2002). *Alzheimer's disease: The costs to U.S. businesses in 2002.* Washington DC: Alzheimer's Association. Retrieved November 26, 2009, from www.alz.org/national/documents/report_alzcosttobusiness.pdf

Koss, E., & Gilmore, G. C. (1998). Environmental interventions and functional ability of AD patients. In B.

Vellas, J. Fitten, & G. Frisoni (Eds.), *Research and practice in Alzheimer's disease* (pp. 185–193). New York: Springer.

Kovach, C. R., & Stearns, S. A. (1994). DSCUs: A study of behavior before and after residence. *Journal of Gerontological Nursing, 29,* 33–39.

Kovach, C. R., Taneli, Y., Dohearty, P., Schlidt, A. M., Cashin, S., & Silva-Smith, A. L. (2004). Effect of the BACE intervention on agitation of people with dementia. *Gerontologist, 44,* 797–806.

Kuhn, D. R., & Mendes de Leon, C. F. (2001). Evaluating an educational intervention with relatives of persons in the early stages of Alzheimer's disease. *Research on Social Work Practice, 11,* 531–548.

Lai, C. K. Y., Chi, I., & Kayser-Jones, J. (2004). A randomized controlled trial of a specific reminiscence approach to promote the well-being of nursing home residents with dementia. *International Psychogeriatrics, 16,* 33–49.

Lantz, M. S., Buchalter, E. N., & McBee, L. (1997). Wellness group: A novel intervention for coping with disruptive behavior in elderly nursing home residents. *Gerontologist, 37*(4), 551–556.

Law, M. (1998). *Client-centered occupational therapy.* Thorofare, NJ: Slack.

Law, M., Baptiste, S., Carswell, A., McColl, M. A., Polatajko, H., & Pollock, N. (2005). *Canadian Occupational Performance Measure.* Toronto, Ontario, Canada: CAOT Publications.

Law, M., & Baum, C. (1998). Evidence-based occupational therapy. *Canadian Journal of Occupational Therapy, 65,* 131–135.

Law, M., Cooper, B., Strong, S., Stewart, D., Rigby, R., & Letts, L. (1996). The Person–Environment–Occupation model: A transactive approach to occupational performance. *Canadian Journal of Occupational Therapy, 63,* 9–23.

Lawler, M. C., & Mattingly, C. F. (1998). The complexities embedded in family-centered care. *American Journal of Occupational Therapy, 52*(4), 259–267.

Lawton, M. P. (1969). Instrumental activities of daily living: Lawton IADL Scale. *Gerontologist, 9,* 179–186.

Lazowski, D., Ecclestone, N., Myers, A., Paterson, D. H., Tudor-Locke, C., Fitzgerald, C., et al. (1999). A randomized outcome evaluation of group exercise programs in long-term care institutions. *Journals of Gerontology: Series A, Biological Sciences and Medical Sciences, 54,* M621.

Lee, H., & Cameron, M. (2004). Respite care for people with dementia and their carers. *Cochrane Database of Systematic Reviews, 1,* 1–18.

Letts, L., Scott, S., Burtney, J., Marshall, L., & McKean, M. (1998). The reliability and validity of the Safety Assessment of Function and the Environment for Rehabilitation (SAFER Tool). *British Journal of Occupational Therapy, 61*(3), 127–132.

Levy, L. L. (1986). A practical guide to the care of the Alzheimer's disease victim: The cognitive disability perspective. *Topics in Geriatric Rehabilitation, 1,* 16–26.

Levy, L. L., & Burns, T. (2005). Cognitive disabilities reconsidered. In N. Katz (Ed.), *Cognition and occupation across the lifespan: Models for intervention in occupational therapy* (2nd ed., pp. 347–385). Bethesda, MD: AOTA Press.

Lewin Group. (2004). *Saving lives, saving money: Dividends for Americans investing in Alzheimer's research.* Washington DC: Alzheimer's Association. Retrieved November 26, 2009, from www.alz.org/national/documents/report_savinglivessavingmoney.pdf

Lezak, M. D., Howieson, D. B., & Loring, D. W. (2004). *Neuropsychological assessment* (4th ed.). New York: Oxford University Press.

Luchsinger, J. A. (2004). Dietary factors and Alzheimer's disease. *Lancet Neurology, 3*(10), 579–587.

Mackintosh, S. F., & Sheppard, L. A. (2005). A pilot falls-prevention programme for older people with dementia from a predominantly Italian background. *Hong Kong Physiotherapy Journal, 23,* 20–26.

Mahendra, N. (2004). Exercise and behavioral management training improves physical health and reduces depression in people with Alzheimer's disease. *Evidence-Based Healthcare, 8*(2), 77.

Mahoney, D. M., Tarlow, B., Jones, R. N., Tennstedt, S., & Kasten, L. (2001). Factors affecting the use of a telephone-based intervention for caregivers of people with Alzheimer's disease. *Journal of Telemedicine and Telecare, 7*(3), 139–148.

Man-Son-Hing, M., Marshall, S. C., Molnar, F. J., & Wilson, K. G. (2007). Systematic review of driving risk and the efficacy of compensatory strategies in persons with dementia. *Journal of the American Geriatrics Society, 55,* 878–884.

Marottoli, R. A., Mendes de Leon, C. F., Glass, T. A., Williams, C. S., Berkman, L. F., et al. (1997). Driving cessation and increased depressive symptoms: Prospective evidence from the New Haven EPESE. *Journal of the American Geriatrics Society, 45,* 202–206.

McCurry, S. M., Gibbons, L. E., Logsdon, R. G., Vitiello, M., & Teri, L. (2003). Training caregivers to change the sleep hygiene practices of patients with dementia: The NITE–AD project. *Journal of the American Geriatrics Society, 51,* 1455–1460.

McCurry, S. M., Gibbons, L. E., Logsdon, R. G., Vitiello, M. V., & Teri, L. (2005). Nighttime insomnia treatment and education for Alzheimer's disease: A randomized controlled trial. *Journal of the American Geriatrics Society, 53,* 793–802.

McGilton, K. S., Rivera, T. M., & Dawson, P. (2003). Can we help persons with dementia find their way in a new environment? *Aging and Mental Health, 7*(5), 363–371.

Mittelman, M. S., Ferris, S. H., Shulman, E., Steingberg, G., & Levin, B. (1996). A family intervention to delay nursing home placement of patients with Alzheimer's disease: A randomized controlled trial. *Journal of the American Medical Association, 276,* 1725–1731.

Mittelman, M. S., Haley, W. E., Clay, O. J., & Roth, D. L. (2006). Improving caregiver well-being delays nursing home placement of patients with Alzheimer disease. *Neurology, 4,* 1592–1599.

Mittelman, M. S., Roth, D. L., Clay, O. J., & Haley, W. E. (2007). Preserving health of Alzheimer caregivers: Impact of a spouse caregiver intervention. *American Journal of Geriatric Psychiatry, 15,* 780–789.

Mittelman, M. S., Roth, D. L., Haley, W. E., & Zarit, S. H. (2004). Effects of a caregiver intervention on negative caregiver appraisals of behavior problems in patients with Alzheimer's disease: Results of a randomized trial. *Journals of Gerontology, 59*(1), P27–P34.

Molnar, F. J., Patel, A., Marshall, S. C., Man-Son-Hing, M., & Wilson, C. G. (2006). Systematic review of the optimal frequency of follow-up in persons with mild dementia who continue to drive. *Alzheimer Disease and Associated Disorders, 20,* 295–297.

Moore, D. P., & Jefferson, J. W. (Eds.). (2004). *Handbook of medical psychiatry* (2nd ed.). St. Louis, MO: Mosby.

Morris, J. C. (1993). The clinical dementia rating (CDR): Current version and scoring rules. *Neurology, 43,* 2412–2414.

Namazi, K. H., & Johnson, B. D. (1992a). The effects of environmental barriers on the attention span of Alzheimer's disease patients. *American Journal of Alzheimer's Care and Related Disorders and Research, 7*(1), 9–15.

Namazi, K. H., & Johnson, B. D. (1992b). Pertinent autonomy for residents with dementias: Modification of the physical environment to enhance independence.

American Journal of Alzheimer's Care and Related Disorders and Research, 7(1), 16–21.

Namazi, K. H., Rosner, T. T., & Calkins, M. P. (1989). Visual barriers to prevent ambulatory Alzheimer's patients from exiting through an emergency door. *Gerontologist, 29*(5), 699–702.

National Alliance for Caregiving. (2004). *Caregiving in the U.S.* (National Alliance for Caregiving and AARP report). Retrieved November 26, 2009, from www.caregiving.org/data/04finalreport.pdf

Nochajski, S. M., Tomita, M. R., & Mann, W. C. (1996). The use and satisfaction with assistive devices by older persons with cognitive impairments: A pilot intervention study. *Topics in Geriatric Rehabilitation, 12*(2), 40–53.

Nolan, B., Mathews, R., & Harrison, M. (2001). Using external memory aids to increase room finding by older adults with dementia. *American Journal of Alzheimer's Disease and Other Dementias, 16,* 251–254.

Nygård, L., & Johansson, M. (2001). The experience and management of temporality in five cases of dementia. *Scandinavian Journal of Occupational Therapy, 8,* 85–95.

Oakley, F., Kielhofner, G., Barris, R., & Reichler, R. K. (1986). The Role Checklist: Development and empirical assessment of reliability. *Occupational Therapy Journal of Research, 6,* 157–169.

Oliver, D., Connelly J. B., Victor, C. R., Shaw, F. E., Whitehead, A., Genc, Y., et al. (2007). Strategies to prevent falls and fractures in hospitals and effect of cognitive impairment: Systematic review and meta-analyses. *British Medical Journal, 334*(7584), 82.

Opie, J., Rosewarne, R., & O'Connor, D. (1999). The efficacy of psychosocial approaches to behaviour disorders in dementia: A systematic literature review. *Australian and New Zealand Journal of Psychiatry, 33,* 789–799.

Orsulic-Jeras, S., Judge, K., & Camp, C. (2000). Montessori-based activities for long-term care residents with advanced dementia: Effects on engagement and affect. *Gerontologist, 40,* 107–111.

Ostaszkiewicz, J., Johnston, L., & Roe, B. (2004a). Habit retraining for the management of urinary incontinence in adults. *Cochrane Database of Systematic Reviews, 2,* CD002801.pub2. doi: 10.1002/14651858 .CD002801.pub2

Ostaszkiewicz, J., Johnston, L., & Roe, B. (2004b). Timed voiding for the management of urinary incontinence in adults. *Cochrane Database of Systematic Reviews, 1,* CD002802.pub2. doi: 10.1002/14651858 .CD002802.pub2

Ott, A., Breteler, M. M., van Harskamp, F., Stijnen, T., & Hofman, A. (1998). Incidence and risk of dementia: The Rotterdam study. *American Journal of Epidemiology, 147,* 574–580.

Ott, B. R., Heindel, W. C., Papandonatos, G. D., Festa, E. C., Davis, J. D., Daiello, L. A., et al. (2008). A longitudinal study of drivers with Alzheimer disease. *Neurology, 70,* 1171–1178.

Pankow, L., Pliskin, N., & Luchins, D. (1996). An optical intervention for visual hallucinations associated with visual impairments and dementia in elderly patients. *Journal of Neuropsychiatry, 8*(1), 88–92.

Passini, R., Pigot, H., Rainville, C., & Tetreault, M. (2000). Way finding in a nursing home for advanced dementia of the Alzheimer's type. *Environment and Behavior, 32*(5), 684–710.

Passini, R., Rainville, C., Marchand, N., & Joanette, Y. (1998). Way finding and dementia: Some research findings and a new look at design. *Journal of Architectural and Planning Research, 15*(2), 133–151.

Peacock, S. C., & Forbes, D. A. (2003). Interventions for caregivers of persons with dementia: A systematic review. *Canadian Journal of Nursing Research, 35*(4), 88–107.

Perkinson, M. A., Berg-Weger, M. L., Carr, D. B., Meuser, T. M., Palmer, J. L., Buckles, V. D., et al. (2005). Driving and dementia of the Alzheimer type: Beliefs and cessation strategies among stakeholders. *Gerontologist, 45,* 676–685.

Pfeffer, R. I., Kurosaki, T. T., Harrah, C. H., Jr., Chance, J. M., & Filos, S. (1982). Measurement of functional activities in older adults in the community. *Journal of Gerontology, 3,* 323–329.

Pinkney, L. (1997). A comparison of the Snoezelen environment and a music relaxation group on the mood and behaviour of patients with senile dementia. *British Journal of Occupational Therapy, 60*(5), 209–212.

Plassman, B. L., Langa, K. M., Fisher, G. G., Heeringa, S. G., Weir, D. R., & Ofstedal, M. B. (2007). Prevalence of dementia in the United States: The aging, demographics, and memory study. *Neuroepidemiology, 29,* 125–132.

Politis, A. M., Vozzella, S., Mayer, L. S., Onyike, C. U., Baker, A. S., & Lyketsos, C. G. (2004). A randomized, controlled, clinical trial of activity therapy for apathy in patients with dementia residing in long-term care. *International Journal of Geriatric Psychiatry, 19*(11), 1087–1094.

Pomeroy, V. M. (1993). The effect of physiotherapy input on mobility skills of elderly people with severe dementing illness. *Clinical Rehabilitation, 7*(2), 163–170.

Pool, J. (2001). Making contact: An activity-based model of care. *Journal of Dementia Care, 9,* 24–26.

Ragland, D. R., Satariano, W. A., & MacLeod, K. E. (2005). Driving cessation and increased depressive symptoms. *Journals of Gerontology: Medical Sciences, 60A,* 399–403.

Rayner, A. V., O'Brien, J. G., & Shoenbachler, B. (2006). Behavior disorders of dementia: Recognition and treatment. *American Family Physicians, 73*(4), 647–652.

Rentz, C. A. (2002). Memories in the making: Outcome-based evaluation of an art program for individuals with dementing illnesses. *American Journal of Alzheimer's Disease and Other Dementias, 17,* 175–181.

Robichaud, L., Hebert, R., & Desrosiers, J. (1994). Efficacy of a sensory integration program on behaviors of inpatients with dementia. *American Journal of Occupational Therapy, 48,* 355–360.

Rogers, J. C., Holm, M. B., Burgio, L. D., Granieri, E., Hsu, C., & Hardin, J. M. (1999). Improving morning care routines of nursing home residents with dementia. *Journal of the American Geriatrics Society, 47*(9), 1049–1057.

Rogers, J. C., Holm, M. B., Chisholm, D., Raina, K. D., & Toto, P. E. (2008, March). *Performance Assessment of Self-care Skills: An observational clinical tool to measure activity performance.* Paper presented at the AOTA Annual Conference & Expo, Long Beach, CA.

Ross, D. G. (1986). *Ross Information Processing Assessment.* Austin, TX: PRO-ED.

Rosswurm, M. A. (1990). Attention-focusing program for persons with dementia. *Clinical Gerontologist, 10*(2), 3–16.

Rovio, S., Kareholt, I., Helkala, E. L., Viitanen, M., Winblad, B., Tuomilehto, J., et al. (2005). Leisure-time physical activity at midlife and the risk of dementia and Alzheimer's disease. *Lancet Neurology, 4*(11), 705–711.

Sackett, D. L., Rosenberg, W. M., Muir Gray, J. A., Haynes, R. B., & Richardson, W. S. (1996). Evidence-based medicine: What it is and what it isn't. *British Medical Journal, 312,* 71–72.

Savage, T., & Matheis-Kraft, C. (2001). Fall occurrence in a geriatric psychiatry setting before and after a fall prevention program. *Journal of Gerontological Nursing, 27,* 49–53.

Scarmeas, N., Luchsinger, J. A., Mayeux, R., & Stern, Y. (2007). Mediterranean diet and Alzheimer disease mortality. *Neurology, 69,* 1084–1093.

Schaber, P. (2002). FIRO model: A framework for family-centered care. *Physical and Occupational Therapy in Geriatrics, 20*(3/4), 1–18.

Schacke, C., & Zank, S. R. (2006). Measuring the effectiveness of adult day care as a facility to support family caregivers of dementia patients. *Journal of Applied Gerontology, 25*(1), 65–81.

Schneider, J. A., Arvanitakis, Z., Bang, W., & Bennett, D. A. (2007). Mixed brain pathologies account for most dementia cases in community-dwelling older persons. *Neurology, 69,* 2197–2204.

Schultz, S. (2009). Theory of occupational adaptation. In E. B. Crepeau, E. S. Cohn, & B. A. Boyt Schell (Eds.), *Willard and Spackman's occupational therapy* (11th ed., pp. 462–475). Baltimore: Lippincott Williams & Wilkins.

Schulz, R., O'Brien, A., Czaja, S., Ory, M., Norris, R., Martire, L. M., et al. (2002). Dementia caregiver intervention research: In search of clinical significance. *Gerontologist, 42*(5), 589–602.

Selzer, M. L., Vinokur, A., & van Rooijen, L. (1975). A self-administered short Michigan Alcohol Screening Test (SMAST). *Journal of Studies of Alcohol, 36*(1), 117–126.

Shaw, G., Kearney, P. J., Vause Earland, T., & Eckhardt, S. M. (2003). Managing dementia-related behaviors. *Home and Community Health Special Interest Section Quarterly, 10*(1), 1–3.

Sherratt, K., Thornton, A., & Hatton, C. (2004). Emotional and behavioural responses to music in people with dementia: An observational study. *Aging and Mental Health, 8*(3), 233–241.

Shobab, L. A. (2005). Cholesterol in Alzheimer's disease. *Lancet Neurology, 4*(12), 841–852.

Shumway-Cook, A., Brauer, S., & Woollacott, M. (2000). Predicting the probability for falls in community-dwelling older adults using the Timed Get Up and Go Test. *Physical Therapy, 80*(9), 896–903.

Skelly, J., & Flint, A. J. (1995). Urinary incontinence associated with dementia. *Journal of the American Geriatrics Society, 43,* 286–294.

Skjerve, A., Bjorvatn, B., & Holsten, F. (2004). Light therapy for behavioural and psychological symptoms of dementia. *International Journal of Geriatric Psychiatry, 19,* 516–522.

Skovdahl, K., Kihlgren, A. L., & Kihlgren, M. (2003). Dementia and aggressiveness: Video-recorded morning care from different care units. *Journal of Clinical Nursing, 12,* 888–898.

Smits, C., de Lange, J., Droes, R., Franka, M., Vernooij-Dassen, M., & Pot, A. (2007). Effects of combined intervention programmes for people with dementia living at home and their caregivers: A systematic review. *International Journal of Geriatric Psychiatry, 22,* 1181–1193.

Snow, L. A., Hovanec, L., & Brandt, J. (2004). A controlled trial of aromatherapy for agitation in nursing home patients with dementia. *Journal of Alternative and Complementary Medicine, 10*(3), 431–37.

Sörensen, S., Pinquart, M., & Duberstein, P. (2002). How effective are interventions with caregivers? An updated meta-analysis. *Gerontologist, 42,* 356–372.

Spector, A., Thorgrtimsen, L., Woods, B., Royan, L., Davies, S., Butterworth, M., et al. (2003). Efficacy of an evidence-based cognitive stimulation therapy program for people with dementia. *British Journal of Psychiatry, 183,* 248–254.

Stav, W. B., Hunt, L. A., & Arbesman, M. (2006). *Occupational therapy practice guidelines for driving and community mobility for older adults.* Bethesda, MD: AOTA Press.

Stenvall, M., Olofsson, B., Lundstroom, M., Englund, U., Borssén, B., Svensson, O., et al. (2007). A multidisciplinary, multifactorial intervention program reduces postoperative falls and injuries after femoral neck fracture. *Osteoporos International, 18,* 167–175.

Swanson, E., Maas, M., & Buckwalter, K. (1994). Alzheimer's residents cognitive and functional measures. *Clinical Nursing, 3,* 27–41.

Tarbell, M. H., Henry, A. D., & Coster, W. J. (2004). Psychometric properties of the scorable self-care evaluation. *American Journal of Occupational Therapy, 58*(3), 324–332.

Teri, L., Gibbons, L. E., McCurry, S. M., Logsdon, R. G., Buchner, D. M., Barlow, W. E., et al. (2003). Exercise and behavioral management training improves physical health and reduces depression in people with Alzheimer's disease. *JAMA, 290,* 2015–2022.

Teri, L., McCurry, S. M., Logsdon, R., & Gibbons, L. E. (2005). Training community consultants to help family members improve dementia care: A randomized controlled trail. *Gerontologist, 45,* 802–811.

Thompson, C., Spilsbury, K., Hall, J., Birks, Y., Barnes, C., & Adamson, J. (2007). Systematic review of information and interventions for caregivers of people with dementia. *BMC Geriatrics, 7,* 18.

Thralow, J. U., & Schauback Reuter, M. J. (1993). Activities of daily living and cognitive levels of function in dementia. *American Journal of Alzheimer's Care and Related Disorders and Research, 8,* 14–19.

Thurman, D. J., Stevens, J. A., & Rao, J. K. (2008). Practice parameter: Assessing patients in a neurology practice for risk of falls. Report of the Quality Standards Committee of the American Academy of Neurology. *Neurology, 70*(6), 473–479.

Tinetti, M. (1991). *Assessment tool—Measures gait and balance as a determinant in risk for falls functional tool box.* McLean, VA: Learn Publications.

Tomaszewski, K. J. (2002). Family altruistic behavior, informal and formal home care, and nursing home entry decisions. (Doctoral dissertation, University of Rochester, New York, 2002). *Dissertation Abstracts International, 63,* 4142. (AAT 3064830)

Topo, P., Jylha, M., & Laine, J. (2002). Can the telephone-using abilities of people with dementia be promoted? An evaluation of a simple-to-use telephone. *Technology and Disability, 14,* 3–13.

Toulotte, C., Fabre, C., Dangremont, B., Lensel, G., & Thevenon, A. (2003). Effects of physical training on the physical capacity of frail, demented patients with a history of falling: A randomized controlled trial. *Age and Ageing, 32,* 67–73.

Trombly, C. A. (1995). Occupation: Purposefulness and meaningfulness as therapeutic mechanisms. *American Journal of Occupational Therapy, 49,* 960–972.

Uc, E. Y., Rizzo, M., Anderson, S. W., Shi, Q., & Dawson, J. D. (2004). Driver route-following and safety errors in early Alzheimer's disease. *Neurology, 63,* 832–1202.

Uc, E. Y., Rizzo, M., Anderson, S. W., Shi, Q., & Dawson, J. D. (2005). Driver landmark and traffic signal identification in early Alzheimer's disease. *Journal of Neurology, Neurosurgery, and Psychiatry 76,* 764–768.

U.S. Bureau of the Census. (2005). *Americans with disabilities: 2005.* Washington, DC: M. W. Brault. Retrieved January 18, 2010, from http://www.census.gov/prod/2008pubs/p70-117.pdf

Vance, D., & Johns, R. (2002). Montessori improved cognitive domains in adults with Alzheimer's disease. *Physical and Occupational Therapy in Geriatrics, 20*(3/4), 19–33.

van Diepen, E., Baillon, S. F., Redman, J., Rooke, N., Spencer, D. A., & Prettyman, R. (2002). A pilot study of the physiological and behavioural effects of Snoezelen in dementia. *British Journal of Occupational Therapy, 65*(2), 61–66.

Vanhanen, M. (2006). Association of metabolic syndrome with Alzheimer's disease: A population-based study. *Neurology, 67*(5), 843–847.

Van Ort, S., & Phillips, L. R. (1995). Nursing intervention to promote functional feeding. *Journal of Gerontological Nursing, 21,* 6–14.

Verghese, J., Lipton, R. B., Vinkers, D. J., Gussekloo, J., Westendorp, R. G. J., Epstein, E. F., et al. (2003). Leisure activities and the risk of dementia in the elderly. *New England Journal of Medicine, 348,* 2508–2516.

Volicer, L., Harper, D. G., Manning, B. C., Goldstein, R., & Satlin, A. (2001). Sundowning and circadian rhythms in Alzheimer's disease. *American Journal of Psychiatry, 158,* 704–711.

Waidmann, T. A. (2003). *Estimates of the risk of long-term care: Assisted living and nursing home facilities.* Washington, DC: Urban Institute Report for the Office of Disability, Aging, and Long-Term Care Policy. Retrieved March 9, 2004, from http://aspe.hhs.gov/daltcp/reports/riskest.pdf

Warner, M. (2000). *The complete guide to Alzheimer's proofing your home.* West Lafayette, IN: Purdue University Press.

Watson, R., & Green, S. (2006). Feeding and dementia: A systematic literature review. *Journal of Advanced Nursing, 54,* 86–93.

Weiner, K. L., Cuncan, P. W., Chandler, J., & Studenski, S. (1992). Functional reach: A marker of physical frailty. *Journal of the American Geriatrics Society, 40,* 203–207.

Whall, A. L., Black, M. E., Groh, C. J., Yankou, D. J., Kupferschmid, B. J., & Foster, M. L. (1997). The effect of natural environments upon agitation and aggression in late-stage dementia patients. *American Journal of Alzheimer's Diseases, 12,* 216–220.

Wilcock, A. A. (2005). Relationship of occupations to health and well-being. In C. H. Christiansen & C. M. Baum (Eds.), *Occupational therapy: Performance, participation and well-being* (pp. 135–165). Thorofare, NJ: Slack.

Wilkinson, N., Srikumar, S., Shaw, K., & Orrell, M. (1998). Drama and movement therapy in dementia: A pilot study. *Arts in Psychotherapy, 25,* 195–201.

Winter, L., & Gitlin, L. N. (2006) Evaluation of a telephone-based support group intervention for female caregivers of community-dwelling individuals with dementia. *American Journal of Alzheimer's Disease and Other Dementias, 21*(6), 391–397.

Wishart, L., Macerollo, J., Loney, P., King, A., Beaumont, L., Browne, G., et al. (2000). "Special steps":

An effective visiting/walking program for persons with cognitive impairment. *Canadian Journal of Nursing Research, 31,* 57–71.

World Health Organization. (2001). *International classification of functioning, disability and health.* Geneva, Switzerland: Author.

Yang, J., Mann, W. C., Nochajski, S., & Tomita, M. R. (1997). Use of assistive devices among elders with cognitive impairment: A follow-up study. *Topics in Geriatric Rehabilitation, 13,* 13–31.

Yesavage, J. A., Brink, T. L., Rose, T. L., Lum, O., Huang, V., Adey, M., et al. (1983). Development and validation of a geriatric depression screening scale: A preliminary report. *Journal of Psychiatric Research 17*(1), 37–49.

■ ■ ■